Use R!

Series Editors:
Robert Gentleman   Kurt Hornik   Giovanni Parmigiani

Use R!

Christian Ritz • Jens Carl Streibig

Nonlinear Regression with R

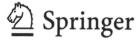 Springer

Christian Ritz
Department of Basic Sciences
and Environment (Statistics)
Faculty of Life Sciences
University of Copenhagen
Thorvaldsensvej 40
DK-1871 Frederiksberg C
Denmark
ritz@life.ku.dk

Jens Carl Streibig
Department of Agriculture and Ecology
(Crop Science)
Faculty of Life Sciences
University of Copenhagen
Hoejbakkegaard Allé 13
DK-2630 Taastrup
Denmark
jcs@life.ku.dk

Series Editors:
Robert Gentleman
Program in Computational Biology
Division of Public Health Sciences
Fred Hutchinson Cancer Research Center
1100 Fairview Ave. N, M2-B876
Seattle, Washington 98109-1024
USA

Kurt Hornik
Department für Statistik und Mathematik
Wirtschaftsuniversität Wien Augasse 2-6
A-1090 Wien
Austria

Giovanni Parmigiani
The Sidney Kimmel Comprehensive Cancer
Center at Johns Hopkins University
550 North Broadway
Baltimore, MD 21205-2011
USA

ISBN: 978-0-387-09615-5   e-ISBN: 978-0-387-09616-2
DOI: 10.1007/978-0-387-09616-2

Library of Congress Control Number: 2008938643

Printed on acid-free paper

springer.com

To Ydun Marie Ritz and in memory of Erik Ritz

Preface

This book is about nonlinear regression analysis with **R**, in particular, how to use the function `nls()` and related functions and methods.

Range of the book

Nonlinear regression may be a confined and narrow topic within statistics. However, the use of nonlinear regression is seen in many applied sciences, ranging from biology to engineering to medicine and pharmacology. Therefore, this book covers a wide range of areas in the examples used. Appendix A lists the disciplines from which data are used in this book.

What not to expect

This book is not a textbook on nonlinear regression. Basic concepts will be briefly introduced, but the reader in need of more explanations will have to consult comprehensive books on nonlinear regression such as Bates and Watts (1988) or Seber and Wild (1989). Instead, this book may be particularly well-suited as an accompanying text, explaining in detail how to carry out nonlinear regression with **R**. However, we also believe that the book is useful as a stand-alone, self-study text for the experimenter or researcher who already has some experience with **R** and at the same time is familiar with linear regression and related basic statistical concepts.

Prerequisites

Experience with **R** at a level corresponding to the first few chapters in Dalgaard (2002) should be sufficient: The user should be acquainted with the basic objects in **R** such as vectors, data frames, and lists, as well as basic plotting and statistics functions for making scatter plots, calculating descriptive statistics, and doing linear regression.

How to read the book

Chapter 2 is essential for getting started on using `nls()`. Section 3.2 and Chapter 4 are at times somewhat technical regarding the use of **R**, whereas Section 6.3 is technical on a statistical level. These parts of the book could be skipped on a first reading.

The **R** extension package `nlrwr` is support software for this book, and it is available at CRAN: http://cran.r-project.org/web/packages/nlrwr/index.html. All datasets and functions used are available upon loading `nlrwr`. All code snippets used in the book are also found in the `scripts` folder that comes with the package. This means that all **R** code snippets shown in this book can be run once the support package `nlrwr` has been installed and loaded. Appendix A provides a list of all datasets used, with a reference to the package where they are found, and Appendix C lists the main functions used in this book together with a package reference.

Acknowledgments

We would like to thank Claire della Vedova and Christian Pipper for proof-reading parts of the book. The first author also wishes to thank the participants of the short course *Non-linear regression with* **R**, held at the Faculty of Life Sciences, University of Copenhagen, in September 2007, for useful comments and suggestions. We are also grateful to Spencer Graves for his valuable comments on an almost final version of the book. All remaining breaches or errors rest solely on the authors.

This volume has benefitted vastly from the many comments and suggestions from the anonymous reviewers of earlier versions. We are also thankful to John Kimmel for his encouragement and guidance throughout this book project.

Finally, we would like to thank the **R** Core Development Team for making all this happen by developing a great open source project. The book has been written using LATEX 2ε and Sweave, yet another powerful invention in the wake of the **R** project.

Copenhagen   *Christian Ritz*
July 2008   *Jens C. Streibig*

Contents

1

Introduction

Throughout this book, we consider a univariate response, say y, that we want to relate to a (possibly multivariate) predictor variable x through a function f. The function f is not completely known, but it is known up to a set of p unknown parameters $\beta = (\beta_1, \ldots, \beta_p)$. We will use various Greek and Latin letters to denote parameters, often using the symbols typically used in the particular models. The relationship between the predictor and the response can be formulated as follows:

$$y = f(x, \beta) \tag{1.1}$$

This book is about the situation where the function f is nonlinear in one or more of the p parameters $\beta_1, \ldots, \beta_p$. In practice, the parameters have to be estimated from the data. Consider a dataset consisting of n pairs $(x_1, y_1), \ldots, (x_n, y_n)$. (The number of parameters occurring in f should be less than the number of observations; that is, $p < n$.) The relationship in Equation (1.1) is for the ideal situation where both the predictor values $x_1, \ldots, x_n$ and the response values $y_1, \ldots, y_n$ are observed without error. In reality, there will be measurement errors that will distort the picture such that none of the pairs $(x_1, y_1), \ldots, (x_n, y_n)$ will fit Equation (1.1) exactly. Therefore, we will assume that the value x_i is predicting the value y_i according to Equation (1.1) apart from some measurement error. In other words, it is more realistic to entertain the idea that the relationship in Equation (1.1) is correct only *on average*. We can formalise this notion by introducing the conditional mean response $E(y_i|x_i)$ (conditional on the predictor value x_i) and recast Equation (1.1) as follows:

$$E(y_i|x_i) = f(x_i, \beta) \tag{1.2}$$

Equation (1.2) reads as follows: Given the predictor value x_i, we will expect the response to be centered around the value $f(x_i, \beta)$. Therefore, we will refer to f as the mean function.

In the formulation above, it is implicitly assumed that the data analyst has some prior knowledge about which kind of function f should be used (at least roughly). Thus nonlinear regression methods are suited for analysing data for which there is an empirically or theoretically established functional relationship between response and predictor.

Each measurement will be distorted by some error related to the measurement process. The observation y_i will differ from the expected mean $E(y_i|x_i)$ by some amount, which we will denote ε_i. The perturbations may be due to minute changes in the measurement process. Therefore, the complete specification of the model of the relationship between the response and the predictor is given by the nonlinear regression model:

$$y_i = E(y_i|x_i) + \varepsilon_i = f(x_i, \beta) + \varepsilon_i \tag{1.3}$$

We will think of the term ε_i as the error term for observation i; that is, the distortion in the response y_i away from the expected value $f(x_i, \beta)$ caused by various unknown sources of variation. The error ε_i will vary from measurement to measurement. Typically, the errors are assumed to be normally distributed with mean 0 and some unknown standard deviation σ that is estimated from the data. We will go into more detail about the assumptions underlying model (1.3) in Chapter 5. We will in this book specify models by means of the mean function involved but implicitly having the complete specification as given in Equation (1.3) in mind. The variables x and y often will be replaced with the actual names being used in a given context and for a given dataset.

Now we will present three examples. The first example is motivating the use of a two-parameter nonlinear regression model. In the second example, a nonlinear regression model involving two predictor variables is introduced. The third example presents a grouped data structure in a nonlinear regression framework.

1.1 A stock-recruitment model

In fisheries biology, there are several theoretical models describing the relationship between the size of the spawning stock (the spawning biomass) and the resulting number of fish (the recruitment). The data frame M.merluccius in the package nlrwr contains three variables: spawn.biomass (the stock), num.fish (the recruitment), and year (which we will not use). Figure 1.1 shows the plot of recruitment versus stock. We may be able to discern an increase that flattens out as spawning biomass increases, but we also notice that there is considerable scatter/variation in the data.

One of these models is the Beverton-Holt model:

$$f\big(S, (\alpha, k)\big) = \frac{\alpha S}{1 + S/k} \tag{1.4}$$

```
> plot(num.fish ~ spawn.biomass,
+     data = M.merluccius, xlab = "Spawning biomass (1000 tonnes)",
+     ylab = "Recruitment (million fish)")
```

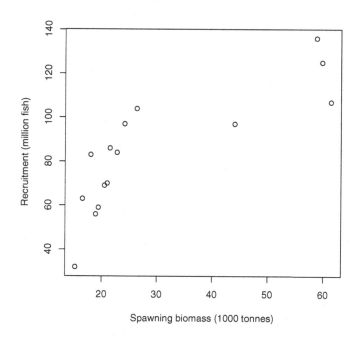

Fig. 1.1. Recruited number of fish plotted against the size of the spawning stock.

The parameter α is the slope at 0, whereas k is the stock resulting in a recruitment halfway between 0 and the upper limit, which is equal to $\alpha \cdot k$. In practice, there is a lot of variability in this kind of data (Cadima, 2003, p. 47), so it is not reasonable to assume that the relationship in Equation (1.4) is deterministic (Carroll and Ruppert, 1988, p. 139), and therefore a nonlinear regression model with the mean function in Equation (1.4) comes into play. We will return to this dataset in Section 7.6.

1.2 Competition between plant biotypes

We want to assess the relative competitive abilities of two biotypes of *Lolium rigidum*. One has developed resistance to glyphosate, and the other is a sensitive wild type (Pedersen et al., 2007). The experimental layout in the greenhouse was an incomplete factorial design. The density of the resistant and sensitive biotypes was based upon the actual density counted after germination (see Fig. 1.2). This sometimes differed from the intended density. The model we use is a hyperbolic model (Jensen, 1993). It describes the competitive ability of the sensitive biotype in relation to the resistant biotype. More specifically, the relationship between biomass per plant of the sensitive biotype (the response) and the densities is described by the function

$$f\big(x, z, (a, b, c)\big) = \frac{a}{1 + b(x + cz)} \qquad (1.5)$$

where x and z are the density per unit area of the sensitive and resistant biotype, respectively. The interpretation of the parameters is:

- a is the theoretical biomass of a plant at zero density.
- b is a measure of the intraspecific competition between plants of the sensitive biotype.
- c is the substitution rate, and it is effectively the exchange rate between the biotypes: If c equals 1, then the two biotypes are equally competitive, and if c is greater than 1, the sensitive biotype is more competitive than the resistant one and vice versa if c is smaller than 1.

The data are in the data frame RScompetition in the package drc. The plot of the data is shown in Fig. 1.2. For the label on the x axis, we use mathematical annotation (see ?plotmath for the details). We use the construct as.numeric(as.factor(RScompetition$z)) to convert the integer values of the variable z in the range 0 to 64 to integer values from 1 to 10, which are suitable as values of the argument pch, which is controlling the plot symbol (Dalgaard, 2002, pp. 8, 173). We will return to this dataset in Subsection 4.4.1.

1.3 Grouped dose-response data

Christensen et al. (2003) describe an experiment that was designed in order to compare the potency of the two herbicide treatments in white mustard plants (*Sinapis alba*).

The data are from a dose-response experiment, which means that a biological stimulus is recorded for a range of doses of some toxic substance. The aim of such experiments is typically to assess the toxicity of the substance applied. The data consist of measurements for the herbicide glyphosate at six different doses and for the herbicide bentazone at seven different doses; for all doses, there are four replicates. The dose is in the unit g/ha and the response is dry matter measured in g/pot. Furthermore, both herbicides have a control of zero dose with eight replicates. The data are available as the data frame S.alba in the package drc. The data frame consists of a total of 68 observations and three variables: the response DryMatter, the predictor Dose, and the factor Herbicide, with two levels (Bentazone and Glyphosate) identifying the two treatments.

```
> plot(biomass ~ x, data = RScompetition,
+     log = "", xlab = Density ~
+         (plants/m^2), ylab = Biomass ~
+         of ~ sensitive ~ biotype ~
+         (g/plant), pch = as.numeric(as.factor(RScompetition$z)))
```

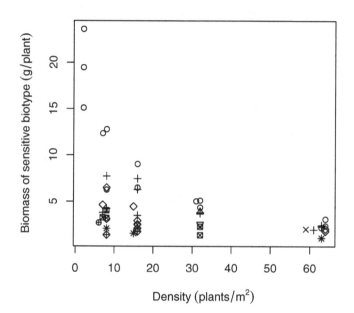

Fig. 1.2. Plot of biomass of sensitive biotype in response to its density. The biomass of the sensitive biotype growing together with the resistant biotype has different symbols.

To get a first impression of the data, we make a plot. As we have two herbicide treatments, we choose a conditional scatter plot using the function xyplot() in the package lattice. The resulting plot is shown in Fig. 1.3 and displays a marked s-shaped or sigmoid curve for each herbicide treatment. One commonly used empirically based model for such dose-response data is the log-logistic model (Streibig et al., 1993) with mean function

$$f\big(\mathrm{dose}, (b, c, d, e)\big) = c + \frac{d - c}{1 + \exp[b\{\log(\mathrm{dose}) - \log(e)\}]} \qquad (1.6)$$

The parameters c and d refer to the lower and upper horizontal asymptotes of the s-shaped curve. The parameter e in model (1.6) is the inflection point of the curve (that is, the point around which it is symmetric on a logarithmic

dose axis), and the parameter b is proportional to the slope at a dose equal to
e. Figure 1.3 reveals that the two curves seem to have roughly the same lower
and upper limits, and they appear to be parallel in the dose range from 20 to
100 g/ha, possibly indicating similar slopes but different inflection points.

```
> xyplot(DryMatter ~ Dose | Herbicide,
+     data = S.alba, scales = list(x = list(log = TRUE)),
+     ylab = "Dry matter (g/pot)",
+     xlab = "Dose (g/ha)")
```

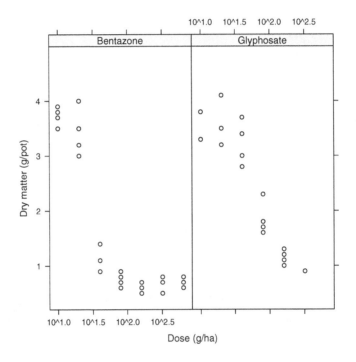

Fig. 1.3. The effect of increasing doses of two herbicide treatments on growth of
white mustard (*Sinapis alba*) plants.

2

Getting Started

In this chapter, we show how to get started fitting nonlinear regression models in **R**. Before getting to **R**, we will provide an ultrabrief summary of the main concepts used when fitting nonlinear regression models (Section 2.1). Much more detailed accounts are provided in the books by Bates and Watts (1988), Seber and Wild (1989), and Huet et al. (2004). Then (in Section 2.2) we will get started using **R**. We focus on the fitting function `nls()`, but in Section 2.3 we introduce another fitting function that may also sometimes be useful in a nonlinear regression context.

2.1 Background

We have predictor values $x_1, \ldots, x_n$, response values $y_1, \ldots, y_n$, and a given mean function f depending on some unknown parameters (in Chapter 1, we already encountered a few examples of mean functions). The parameter estimates are determined as the parameters providing the best fit of the mean function f to the observations $y_1, \ldots, y_n$ obtained by minimisation of the residual sums of squares (RSS) with respect to β:

$$\text{RSS}(\beta) = \sum_{i=1}^{n} \left(y_i - f(x_i, \beta) \right)^2 \tag{2.1}$$

The minimisation of RSS is often referred to as minimising the least-squares criterion or least-squares estimation, and the solution to the minimisation problem is the least-squares parameter estimates, which we denote $\hat{\beta}$. These estimates are the β values (within the domain of all β values that are meaningful for a given mean function f) that make RSS as small as possible. In other words, the global minimum of $\text{RSS}(\beta)$ is attained for $\beta = \hat{\beta}$. In contrast to linear regression (Dalgaard, 2002, pp. 95–96), the minimisation of RSS will in general be a nonlinear problem due to the nonlinearity of f, and therefore numerical optimisation methods are needed. These methods are iterative procedures that will ideally approach the optimal parameter values in a stepwise manner. At each step, the algorithms determine the new parameter values based on the data, the model, and the current parameter values. By far the most common algorithm for estimation in nonlinear regression is the Gauss-Newton method, which relies on linear approximations to the nonlinear mean function at each step. For more details and explanations, see, for example, Bates and Watts (1988, pp. 32–66), Seber and Wild (1989, pp. 21–89), or Weisberg (2005, pp. 234–237). The numerical optimisation methods are not perfect. Two common complications when using them are:

- how to start the procedure and how to choose the initial/starting parameter value
- how to ensure that the procedure reached the global minimum rather than a local minimum

These two issues are interrelated. If the initial parameter values are sufficiently close to the optimal parameter values, then the procedure will usually get closer and closer to the optimal parameter value (the algorithm is said to converge) within a few steps. Therefore, it is very important to provide sensible starting parameter values. Poorly chosen starting values on the other hand will often lead the procedures astray so no useful model fit is obtained. If lack of convergence persists regardless of the choice of starting values, then it typically indicates that the model in its present form is not appropriate for the data at hand (if possible, you could try fitting a related but simpler model).

As the solutions to nonlinear regression problems are numeric, they may differ as a consequence of different algorithms, different implementations of the same algorithm (for example, different criteria for declaring convergence or whether or not first derivatives are computed numerically or explicit expressions are provided), different parameterisations, or different starting values. However, the resulting parameter estimates often will not differ much. If there are large discrepancies, then it may possibly indicate that a simpler model should be preferred.

Once the parameter estimates $\hat{\beta}$ are found, the estimate of the residual variance σ^2 is obtained as the minimum value of RSS (attained when parameter estimates are inserted) divided by the degrees of freedom $(n-p)$, giving the estimate $s^2 = \frac{\text{RSS}(\hat{\beta})}{n-p}$ (Fox, 2002). The residual standard error is then s.

2.2 Getting started with nls()

In this section, we will introduce the key player in this book, the model fitting function nls() (Bates and Chambers, 1992), which comes with the standard installation of **R** (in the package stats). We go through an example showing how to fit a model, how to obtain parameter estimates, predictions, and summary measures, and how to make plots of the fitted mean function or regression curve.

2.2.1 Introducing the data example

We consider data from an experiment on N uptake reported by Cedergreen and Madsen (2002), where the predictor variable is the initial substrate concentration and the response variable is the uptake rate. In this type of experiment, it is anticipated that the uptake will increase as the concentration increases, approaching a horizontal asymptote. The data are available as the data frame L.minor. To get a first impression, we display the data frame by typing the name of the dataset at the command line.

```
> L.minor
```

```
       conc       rate
1    2.856829   14.58342
2    5.005303   24.74123
3    7.519473   31.34551
4   22.101664   72.96985
5   27.769976   77.50099
6   39.198025   96.08794
7   45.483269   96.96624
8  203.784238  108.88374
```

The data frame L.minor contains eight observations. The response is named rate and the predictor is named conc.

A graphical display of the dataset can be obtained using the default plot method. The first argument is a model formula giving the response on the left-hand side of the ~ symbol and the predictor on the right-hand side. As the second argument, we specify the data frame where the predictor and response are found. Finally, we provide informative labels for both the x and y axes of the plot.

The resulting plot is shown in Fig. 2.1. The steep ascent for small concentrations and the ensuing approach towards a horizontal asymptote are easily seen in Fig. 2.1.

2.2.2 Model fitting

Kinetics data such as those in L.minor are often described by the Michaelis-Menten model (Bates and Watts, 1988, p. 33). The model describes the uptake rate as a function of the substrate concentration through the model

$$f\big(\text{concentration}, (K, V_m)\big) = \frac{V_m \cdot \text{concentration}}{K + \text{concentration}} \tag{2.2}$$

```
> plot(rate ~ conc, data = L.minor,
+       ylab = "Uptake rate (weight/h)",
+       xlab = Substrate ~ concentration ~
+            (mmol ~ m^-3))
```

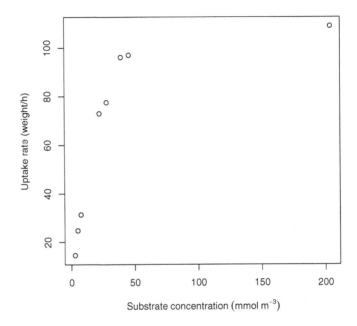

Fig. 2.1. Velocity curve showing uptake rate as a function of substrate concentration based on the data frame `L.minor`.

using two parameters: K and V_m. In a more abstract formulation, the same Michaelis-Menten model can be written as

$$f\left(x, (K, V_m)\right) = \frac{V_m x}{K + x} \qquad (2.3)$$

with x and y playing the roles of the predictor and response, respectively. The mean function f is the right-hand side in Equation (2.3); that is, $f\left(x, (K, V_m)\right) = \frac{V_m x}{K+x}$. At concentration 0, the model predicts a rate equal to 0, and as the substrate concentration becomes larger and larger, the rate approaches from below the upper limit or horizontal asymptote V_m. The parameter K is the substrate concentration where the rate is halfway between 0 and V_m.

Fitting the Michaelis-Menten model to the data frame `L.minor` can be done conveniently using `nls()`.

```
> L.minor.m1 <- nls(rate ~ Vm * conc/(K +
+     conc), data = L.minor, start = list(K = 20,
+     Vm = 120), trace = TRUE)

624.3282 :   20 120
244.5460 :   15.92382 124.57148
234.5198 :   17.25299 126.43877
234.3595 :   17.04442 125.96181
234.3533 :   17.08574 126.04671
234.3531 :   17.07774 126.03016
234.3531 :   17.07930 126.03338
234.3531 :   17.07899 126.03276
```

The first argument, rate~Vm*conc/(K+conc), is the model formula, where ~ is used to relate the response, rate, on the left-hand side to the expression for the mean function, Vm*conc/(K+conc), which is explicitly formulated on the right-hand side. The specification of the mean function involves both the predictor (conc) and the parameters (K and V_m), so parameters have to be named explicitly, in contrast to the linear regression specification in lm() (Dalgaard, 2002, pp. 95–110). Alternatively, we could have supplied a previously defined mean function (defined as an **R** function) instead of the expression Vm*conc/(K+conc) (see Exercise 2.2). Note that in the formula the parameters in the supplied mean function are identified as the names not corresponding to variables in the data frame or the search path and not corresponding to mathematical operations and functions.

In the second argument (data), the data frame containing the response (rate) and the predictor (conc) is specified. In order to initiate the estimation algorithm, we need to supply starting values for the parameters.

We use the argument start to supply the starting values. Having in mind the interpretation of the model parameters given in Subsection 2.2.1, we can read off from Fig. 2.1 an approximate upper limit at a rate of 120, and the rate is roughly halfway (that is, at $120/2 = 60$) around a concentration of 20. The argument trace controls whether or not the parameter values at each step in the iterative estimation procedure should be displayed. We see that the parameter values rapidly stabilise, indicating that the initial values were good guesses.

It is useful to report the value of $\mathrm{RSS}(\hat{\beta})$, or equivalently the estimated residual standard error or variance, as a summary measure of the model fit. Such a summary measure is useful for comparing different model fits (based on different mean functions or software) to the same dataset (see Exercise 2.5) or even for comparing different models (see Section 7.6). To obtain the minimum value of RSS, the value $\mathrm{RSS}(\hat{V}_m, \hat{K})$, we can use the deviance method.

```
> deviance(L.minor.m1)
```

```
[1] 234.3531
```

Another summary measure of the fit that is sometimes reported is the value of the logarithm of the likelihood function, evaluated at the parameter estimates. The likelihood function is closely related to RSS, defined in Equation (2.1), and is defined as follows:

$$L(\beta, \sigma^2) = \frac{1}{(2\pi\sigma^2)^{n/2}} \exp\left\{ -\frac{\text{RSS}(\beta)}{2\sigma^2} \right\}$$

The parameter estimates $\hat{\beta}$ are the parameters that maximise L as a function in β, but this is equivalent to minimising RSS as a function in β. The resulting maximum value of the likelihood function is

$$L(\hat{\beta}, \hat{\sigma}^2) = \frac{1}{(2\pi\text{RSS}(\hat{\beta})/n)^{n/2}} \exp(-n/2) \tag{2.4}$$

where we use the estimate $\hat{\sigma}^2 = \frac{n-p}{n}s^2$. Fox (2002) and Huet et al. (2004) provide more details. The maximum value of the logarithm-transformed likelihood function, which is often simply referred to as the log likelihood function, can be obtained using the logLik method.

```
> logLik(L.minor.m1)
```

```
'log Lik.' -24.86106 (df=3)
```

In addition to the value of the log likelihood function, the number of parameters $(p + 1)$ is shown.

We can use the coef method to list the parameter estimates:

```
> coef(L.minor.m1)
```

```
        K         Vm
 17.07899 126.03276
```

The output is simply a vector of the parameter estimates, nothing else. For a more detailed summary of the model fit, we can use the summary method.

```
> summary(L.minor.m1)
```

```
Formula: rate ~ Vm * conc/(K + conc)
```

```
Parameters:
    Estimate Std. Error t value Pr(>|t|)
K     17.079      2.953   5.784  0.00117 **
Vm   126.033      7.173  17.570 2.18e-06 ***
---
Signif. codes:  0 '***' 0.001 '**' 0.01 '*' 0.05 '.' 0.1 ' ' 1
```

```
Residual standard error: 6.25 on 6 degrees of freedom
```

```
Number of iterations to convergence: 7
Achieved convergence tolerance: 8.144e-06
```

The specified model formula is displayed at the top. Then the parameter estimates and related quantities are shown. The parameter estimates are found in the first column: The horizontal asymptote is attained at 17.1, and the substrate concentration resulting in an increase from 0 to $V_m/2$ is 126. The second column contains the estimated standard errors of the parameter estimates, which are the square roots of the diagonal elements in the estimated variance-covariance matrix

$$\widehat{\text{var}}(\hat{\beta}) = s^2 \hat{B} \tag{2.5}$$

where $\hat{B}$ is the inverse of the matrix of second derivatives of the log likelihood function as a function of β evaluated at the parameter estimates $\beta = \hat{\beta}$. This matrix is often called the Hessian. In nls(), the Hessian matrix is calculated using numeric approximation. Note that different approximations of the Hessian matrix may lead to (usually) small differences in estimated standard errors. Columns 3 and 4 contain t-tests for testing the hypothesis that the parameter is 0. We will discuss hypothesis testing in more detail in Chapter 7, but for the time being we note that these hypotheses are not always relevant to consider. Finally, the estimated residual standard error can also be read directly off the summary output ($s = 6.25$) together with the corresponding degrees of freedom ($n - p = 6$). Finally, some details on the estimation procedure are reported:

- number of iterations needed for the estimation algorithm (here seven iterations (eight evaluations) were used, but we already know this from the trace output)
- tolerance at the final step (difference between the last two evaluations)

The fitted Michaelis-Menten regression curve is given by the following expression:

$$\text{rate} = \frac{17.1 \cdot \text{concentration}}{126 + \text{concentration}} \tag{2.6}$$

2.2.3 Prediction

Equation (2.6) can be used for calculating predicted values. For given concentrations that are supplied, the resulting predicted rates can be determined using Equation (2.6). If we use the same concentrations present in the dataset L.minor, then we get the fitted values, but in all other cases we use the model fit to interpolate between or extrapolate beyond the original concentrations in the dataset, and the resulting values are called predicted values. The fitted values are the model-based predictions for the predictor values in the dataset considered, and they play an important role in constructing model diagnostics such as residual plots. The fitted values can be obtained directly from the nls() fit using the fitted method, with the model fit as the only argument. For instance, the fitted values from the model fit L.minor.m1 are obtained in the following way:

```
> fitted(L.minor.m1)

[1]   18.06066   28.56474   38.52679
[4]   71.09461   78.03806   87.78424
[7]   91.62683 116.28685
attr(,"label")
[1] "Fitted values"
```

In general, prediction can be viewed as follows. For N specified predictor values $x_{01}, \ldots, x_{0N}$, we want to predict the values $f(x_{01}, \hat{\beta}), \ldots, f(x_{0N}, \hat{\beta})$. To do this in **R**, we need to supply both the model fit and the data frame containing the predictor values $x_{01}, \ldots, x_{0N}$. Let us return to the model fit L.minor.m1. First, we define a vector of predictor values (that is, concentrations) for which we want to get predictions.

```
> concVal <- with(L.minor, seq(min(conc),
+     max(conc), length.out = 10))
```

Explanation: Throughout this book, we will use the function with() whenever we want to manipulate with variables inside a data frame. The first argument to with() is the data frame, whereas the second argument is whatever manipulation we want to do (here it is to use the function seq() for generating a sequence of numbers). We want ten predictions based on equidistantly spaced concentrations within the range of concentrations in the original dataset L.minor. Therefore we use the function seq to generate a sequence of concentrations, starting at the minimum concentration in the dataset (obtained using min(conc)) and ending at the maximum concentration in the dataset (max(conc)). In total, ten values are generated (governed by the argument length.out). The concentrations generated are stored in the vector concVal.

The predictions based on the concentrations in concVal are obtained using the predict method.

```
> predict(L.minor.m1, data.frame(conc = concVal))

[1]   18.06066   75.09908   92.70509
[4] 101.26607 106.32776 109.67157
[7] 112.04518 113.81733 115.19094
[10] 116.28685
```

Note that inside the data frame we have to assign the same name to the generated concentrations as is used for the concentrations in the dataset L.minor, which is conc. Using the predict method without supplying a data frame results in the same output as obtained from the fitted method. We will use the predict method in the next subsection because predict is useful for constructing plots.

2.2.4 Making plots

In order to create a plot of the original data with the fitted regression curve superimposed, we have to proceed through a few steps. The original data are plotted using the default plot method.

```
> plot(rate ~ conc, data = L.minor,
+     ylim = c(10, 130), ylab = "Uptake rate (weight/h)",
+     xlab = Substrate ~ concentration ~
+         (mmol ~ m^-3))
> lines(L.minor$conc, fitted(L.minor.m1))
```

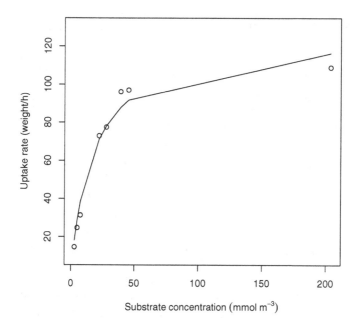

Fig. 2.2. Rate versus substrate concentration in L.minor plotted together with a crude approximation to the fitted Michaelis-Menten regression curve.

We specify the graphical argument ylim in plot to ensure a sufficiently large plot window encompassing both the original data and the entire fitted regression curve. The function `lines()` connects the fitted values for each concentration in the dataset `L.minor` with line segments (linear interpolation). The result in Fig. 2.2 is a crude approximation to the fitted regression curve.

In order to get a nicer (smoother) plot of the estimated regression curve, we need to define a finer grid on the x axis. Figure 2.3 shows the original data in `L.minor` plotted together with a smooth approximation of the fitted regression curve, which is obtained by first generating a sequence of 100 equally spaced concentrations (using the function `seq()`) between the minimum and maximum concentrations in the dataset `L.minor` (using the functions `min()` and `max()`). These 100 concentrations are stored in the vector named `concVal`. The use of the function `with()` with first argument `L.minor` avoids having to make explicit reference to the data frame `L.minor` every time we consider a variable inside the data frame (we need to use `conc` twice), and this way the resulting **R** statement is shortened.

The estimated horizontal asymptote has been added using the function `abline()`, which can be used to add arbitrary lines (horizontal, vertical, or determined by intercept and slope) to a plot (Dalgaard, 2002, p. 99). Here we specify a horizontal line (argument `h`) at `coef(L.minor.m1)[2]`, which is the second component in the vector of parameter estimates, the parameter estimate of V_m. A dashed line type is requested by the argument `lty = 2` (Murrell, 2006, pp. 59–61). The agreement between the data and the model appears to be acceptable, although the estimated horizontal asymptote is overshooting a bit.

2.2.5 Illustrating the estimation

The RSS function for the Michaelis-Menten model based on the dataset `L.minor` is defined as follows using Equation (2.1):

$$\text{RSS}(K, V_m) = \sum_{i=1}^{8} \left(\text{rate}_i - \frac{V_m \cdot \text{concentration}_i}{K + \text{concentration}_i} \right)^2$$

So for a grid of pairs of K and V_m values, we can calculate the values $\text{RSS}(K, V_m)$, and it can be visualised by means of a contour plot connecting pairs of K and V_m values that result in the same value of $\text{RSS}(K, V_m)$. This approach is possible for any model with at most two parameters ($p = 2$). The function `nlsContourRSS()` in the package `nlstools` constructs an object containing all the information needed for making the contour plot. The only argument that we need to supply to `nlsContourRSS()` is the model fit for which a contour plot should be generated. The following line generates a contour plot object based on the model fit `L.minor.m1`.

```
> L.minor.m1con <- nlsContourRSS(L.minor.m1)
```

The corresponding `plot` method is then applied to show the contour plot. Apart from the model fit we specify, the absence of most colours in the plot

```
> plot(rate ~ conc, data = L.minor,
+     ylim = c(10, 130), ylab = "Uptake rate (weight/h)",
+     xlab = Substrate ~ concentration ~
+         (mmol ~ m^-3))
> concVal <- with(L.minor, seq(min(conc),
+     max(conc), length.out = 100))
> lines(concVal, predict(L.minor.m1,
+     newdata = data.frame(conc = concVal)))
> abline(h = coef(L.minor.m1)[2],
+     lty = 2)
```

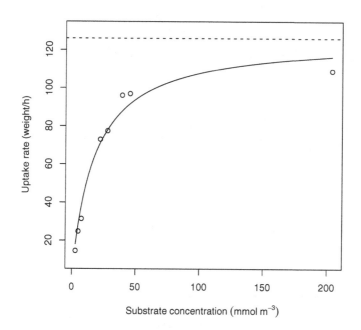

Fig. 2.3. Rate versus substrate concentration in L.minor plotted together with a smooth version of the fitted Michaelis-Menten regression curve. The estimated horizontal asymptote is the dashed line.

(col = FALSE), and we decide to display ten contour levels. The resulting contour plot is shown in Fig. 2.4. Each contour level corresponds to all pairs of parameter values (K, V_m) producing the same value of RSS. In addition to the ten contour levels, a dashed contour line defines a region that corresponds to a 95% confidence region of the two parameters (see ?nlsContourRSS for more details). The narrowing contour lines clearly indicate the approximate location of the parameter estimates.

```
> plot(L.minor.m1con, col = FALSE,
+    nlev = 10)
```

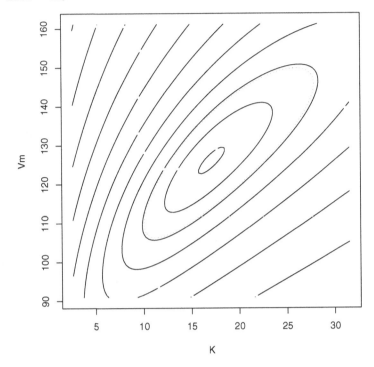

Fig. 2.4. Contour plot of the residual sums-of-squares function RSS(K, V_m) for the Michaelis-Menten model fitted to the dataset **L.minor**. The region encompassed by the dashed contour is a 95% confidence region (see Chapter 7 for more details).

2.3 Generalised linear models

In this section, we briefly present another fitting function that sometimes may be useful in relation to nonlinear regression.

Some nonlinear regression models can be treated as generalised linear models, which are a collection of statistical models where it is possible to transform the mean function in such a way that a linear model is recovered on some transformed scale (McCullagh and Nelder, 1989, Chapter 1). One advantage of using a generalised linear model is that there is typically no need to specify starting values.

Let us once more return to the dataset **L.minor** and the Michaelis-Menten model. The mean function can be rewritten as follows (which works because we assume all predictor values are positive):

$$f\big(x, (K, V_m)\big) = \frac{1}{\frac{1}{V_m} + \frac{K}{V_m}\frac{1}{x}} = \frac{1}{\tilde{\beta}_0 + \tilde{\beta}_1\frac{1}{x}}$$

Thus the reciprocal mean function looks like

$$\frac{1}{f(x, (K, V_m))} = \tilde{\beta}_0 + \tilde{\beta}_1 \frac{1}{x}$$

which is a linear regression formulation in $1/x$ (the so-called linear predictor) with intercept parameter $\tilde{\beta}_0 = 1/V_m$ and slope parameter $\tilde{\beta}_1 = K/V_m$. Consequently the Michaelis-Menten model can be viewed as a generalised linear model with the inverse or reciprocal function as the link function between the original and transformed scales for the mean (McCullagh and Nelder, 1989; Nelder, 1991, Chapter 8). Going to the generalised linear model formulation changed the parameterisation, so we will need to do some extra work in order to retrieve the original parameters K and V_m from the generalised linear model fit.

The main model fitting function in **R** for generalised linear models is glm(), which is explained in more detail by Venables and Ripley (2002a, Chapter 7) and Dalgaard (2002, Chapter 11). We can fit the model to the dataset L.minor as follows:

```
> L.minor.m4 <- glm(rate ~ I(1/conc),
+     data = L.minor, family = gaussian("inverse"))
```

The first argument is the model formula rate~I(1/conc), specifying the response and the linear regression formulation. We use the function I() whenever we manipulate with a predictor on the right-hand side of a model formula. This way the manipulation is protected and not interpreted in relation to the usual rules governing model specification (Dalgaard, 2002, Chapter 10). The transformation to be applied to the linear predictor ("inverse") and the distribution assumed (gaussian) are specified in the argument family. The resulting summary output is shown below.

```
> summary(L.minor.m4)

Call:
glm(formula = rate ~ I(1/conc), family = gaussian("inverse"),
    data = L.minor)

Deviance Residuals:
   Min      1Q   Median      3Q     Max
-7.403  -4.663   -2.007   2.741   8.304

Coefficients:
            Estimate Std. Error t value Pr(>|t|)
(Intercept) 0.0079344  0.0004516  17.570 2.18e-06 ***
I(1/conc)   0.1355123  0.0173574   7.807 0.000233 ***
---
Signif. codes:  0 '***' 0.001 '**' 0.01 '*' 0.05 '.' 0.1 ' ' 1
```

(Dispersion parameter for gaussian family taken to be 39.05854)

Null deviance: 9427.92   on 7   degrees of freedom
Residual deviance: 234.35   on 6   degrees of freedom
AIC: 55.722

Number of Fisher Scoring iterations: 7

The output is quite similar to what `nls()` produces. Dalgaard (2002, Chapter 11) provides a detailed explanation for all components in the output.

Exercises

2.1. Fit the exponential model

$$f\big(x, (b, y_0)\big) = y_0 \exp(x/b)$$

with parameters b (controlling the rate of change) and y_0 (average response level at $x = 0$) to the dataset `RGRcurve`. Make a plot of the original data with the estimated curve superimposed. Comment on the plot.

2.2. The mean function of the Michaelis-Menten model can be defined as the following **R** function:

```
> MMfct <- function(conc, K, Vm) {
+     Vm * conc/(K + conc)
+ }
```

Use the function `MMfct()` to fit the Michaelis-Menten model to the dataset `L.minor` introduced in Subsection 2.2.1.

2.3. Use the function `plotfit()` for plotting the data in `L.minor` together with the fitted Michaelis-Menten regression curve based on the model fit `L.minor.m1`. Note that `plotfit()` only works for model fits involving a one-dimensional predictor without any grouping structure.

2.4. Venables and Ripley (2002a) consider an extension of the exponential model introduced in Exercise 2.1. The extended model involves three parameters; the additional parameter describes the lower, horizontal asymptote of the regression curve. The extended exponential model is given by the function

$$f\big(x, (\beta_1, \beta_2, \beta_3)\big) = \beta_1 2^{-x/\beta_2} + \beta_3$$

All three parameters have a biological interpretation: β_1 is the final weight, β_2 is the time where the weight is halfway between the initial weight and final weight β_1, and β_3 is the weight loss.

   Fit the extended exponential model to the dataset `wtloss` found in the package `MASS` by guessing appropriate starting values.

.

2.5. As seen in Section 1.1, the Beverton-Holt model can be used to describe stock-recruitment relationships. The model is a reparameterisation of another model used in Chapter 2. Which model? Use `nls()` to fit this model to the dataset `M.merluccius`. Plot the data together with the fitted regression curve.

In Cadima (2003, p. 131), the reported parameter estimates are $\hat{\alpha} = 4.91$ and $\hat{k} = 45.39$. How does this agree with the parameter estimates obtained from the `nls()` fit? Add the regression curve based on Cadima's parameters to the plot showing the `nls()` fit. Which model fit is best?

3

Starting Values and Self-starters

This chapter is about how to find appropriate starting values and how to use self-starter functions. We present several techniques for finding initial parameter values in Section 3.1. The use of self-starter functions, which are functions that substitute for a manual search for starting values, is introduced in Section 3.2.

3.1 Finding starting values

Finding starting values for the parameters by "eye-balling" appeared to work fine in the previous section. This way of guessing the initial parameter values is the most common approach for obtaining starting values. It may require some skill or experience from previous analyses to come up with a successful guess. On the other hand, simply trying out a range of parameter values will sometimes suffice. If the mean function in the nonlinear regression model has parameters with an interpretation, then it may be easy to read off starting values from a plot of the data. If this is not the case, then it may be useful

- to jointly explore the data and the model function graphically
- to search for good initial parameter values

In the following two subsections, we will focus on these strategies.

3.1.1 Graphical exploration

Typically some parameters have a subject-specific (e.g., biological, chemical, or physical) interpretation, whereas the remaining parameters do not.

The dataset Chwirut2 in the package NISTnls contains measurements from an experiment examining how ultrasonic response depends on the metal distance, and it stems from an NIST study involving ultrasonic calibration (NIST (National Institute of Standards and Technology), 1979). Data are shown in Fig. 3.1 and seem to exhibit some kind of exponential decay.

```
> library(NISTnls)
> plot(y ~ x, data = Chwirut2, xlab = "Metal distance",
+     ylab = "Ultrasonic response")
```

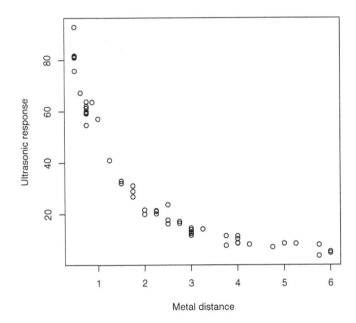

Fig. 3.1. Plot of the dataset `Chwirut2` showing how ultrasonic response depends on metal distance.

The model suggested by NIST (National Institute of Standards and Technology) (1979) for this dataset is an exponential decay model where the response y (ultrasonic response) is related to the predictor x (metal distance) through the mean function

$$f\big(x, (\beta_1, \beta_2, \beta_3)\big) = \frac{\exp(-\beta_1 x)}{\beta_2 + \beta_3 x} \tag{3.1}$$

For $x = 0$, the model gives the value $1/\beta_2$, and thus β_2 can be taken to be the reciprocal of the response value closest to the y axis, which is roughly $1/100 = 0.01$. The two remaining parameters do not have a similar simple interpretation. Therefore, we want to explore graphically how the mean function f is situated for different choices of the parameters.

First, the mean function in Equation (3.1) is defined.

```
> expFct <- function(x, beta1, beta2,
+     beta3) {
```

```
+        exp(-beta1 * x)/(beta2 + beta3 *
+        x)
+ }
```

Next we plot the data and add the curve for a given choice of parameter values on top of the plot using the function curve() (Dalgaard, 2002, p. 31). In Fig. 3.2, the resulting explorative plot is shown. For our initial choice of parameter values, which are $\beta_1 = 1$, $\beta_2 = 0.01$, and $\beta_3 = 1$, the mean function is hardly visible, lying slightly above the x axis except for those close to $x = 0$.

```
> plot(y ~ x, data = Chwirut2, xlab = "Metal distance",
+        ylab = "Ultrasonic response",
+        ylim = c(0, 100))
> curve(expFct(x, beta1 = 1, beta2 = 0.01,
+        beta3 = 1), add = TRUE)
```

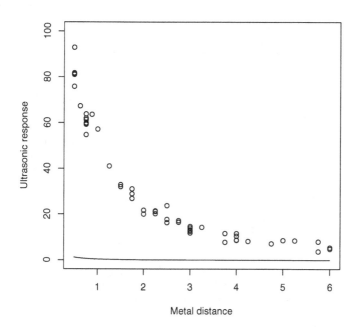

Fig. 3.2. Explorative plot showing the mean function for a given configuration of the parameter values ($\beta_1 = 1$, $\beta_2 = 0.01$, and $\beta_3 = 1$) together with the data from the dataset Chwirut2.

So our initial choice of parameter values was not great. Therefore let us try out four other configurations, $(0.1, 0.01, 1)$, $(0.1, 0.01, 0.1)$, $(0.1, 0.01, 0.01)$, and $(0.2, 0.01, 0.01)$, where we only make a change in one of the parameters at a time. The four resulting explorative plots are shown in Fig. 3.3. They are produced using curve(). The argument lty in curve() is used to obtain different line types for the four curves.

```
> plot(y ~ x, data = Chwirut2, xlab = "Metal distance",
+     ylab = "Ultrasonic response",
+     ylim = c(0, 100))
> curve(expFct(x, beta1 = 0.1, beta2 = 0.01,
+     beta3 = 1), add = TRUE, lty = 2)
> curve(expFct(x, beta1 = 0.1, beta2 = 0.01,
+     beta3 = 0.1), add = TRUE, lty = 3)
> curve(expFct(x, beta1 = 0.1, beta2 = 0.01,
+     beta3 = 0.01), add = TRUE,
+     lty = 4)
> curve(expFct(x, beta1 = 0.2, beta2 = 0.01,
+     beta3 = 0.01), add = TRUE,
+     lty = 1)
```

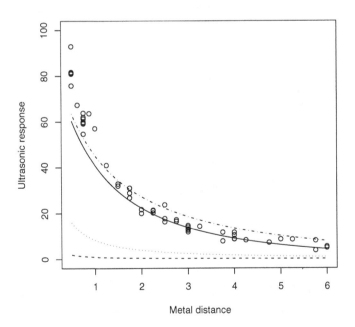

Fig. 3.3. Four explorative plots to see how the mean function varies with the parameter values: long-dashed $(0.1, 0.01, 1)$, short-dashed $(1, 0.01, 0.1)$, long–short-dashed $(0.1, 0.01, 0.01)$ and solid $(0.2, 0.01, 0.01)$.

We see from Fig. 3.3 how the chosen parameter values result in a mean function lying closer and closer to the data. In practice, you may need more than just a few tries to get the mean function close to the data (see Exercise 3.1).

The parameter values producing the solid curve in Fig. 3.3 seem to roughly fit the data, so let us try to use these parameter values as starting values.

```
> Chwirut2.m1 <- nls(y ~ expFct(x,
+      beta1, beta2, beta3), data = Chwirut2,
+      start = list(beta1 = 0.2, beta2 = 0.01,
+          beta3 = 0.01))
```

We get no errors, and it seems that the estimation algorithm converged. The summary output of the model fit is shown below.

```
> summary(Chwirut2.m1)

Formula: y ~ expFct(x, beta1, beta2, beta3)

Parameters:
        Estimate Std. Error t value Pr(>|t|)
beta1 0.1665753  0.0383032   4.349 6.56e-05 ***
beta2 0.0051653  0.0006662   7.753 3.54e-10 ***
beta3 0.0121501  0.0015304   7.939 1.81e-10 ***
---
Signif. codes:  0 '***' 0.001 '**' 0.01 '*' 0.05 '.' 0.1 ' ' 1

Residual standard error: 3.172 on 51 degrees of freedom

Number of iterations to convergence: 5
Achieved convergence tolerance: 4.688e-06
```

Indeed, the estimation algorithm converged in five steps, producing parameter estimates that seem reasonable, as they are quite close to the initial values that we provided and that already seemed to provide an acceptable fit as judged from Fig. 3.3. Note that the parameter values used in the first explorative plot in Fig. 3.2 will not work, but instead they will result in nls() terminating with an error message.

3.1.2 Searching a grid

In case you have an idea about the range within which the parameter estimates should be lying, it can be useful to carry out a grid search: to evaluate the residual sums-of-squares function $\text{RSS}(\beta)$ for a coarse grid based on the ranges supplied for the parameters and then to choose as starting values the parameter values that yield the smallest value of $\text{RSS}(\beta)$.

Consider again the dataset Chwirut2 and the mean function defined in Equation (3.1). Without having any idea about the range of β_1 and β_3 (we know that β_2 is roughly around 0.01) apart from the fact that they are positive numbers, we could search through a rather small grid from 0.1 to 1 at steps of size 0.1 for both parameters. Thus we want to search through a grid with the following ranges for the three parameters:

β_1: 0.1 to 1
β_2: 0.01 (fixed at one value)
β_3: 0.1 to 1

We approximate the ranges listed above for the parameters β_1 and β_3 by generating two vectors of parameter values using the function seq() (Dalgaard, 2002, Chapter 1). The result of seq(0.1, 1, by=0.1) is a vector of length 10 (the numbers from 0.1 to 1 in steps of 0.1). We define the grid of all combinations or triples of the elements in the three vectors seq(0.1, 1, by=0.1) for β_1, c(0.01) for β_2 (a vector with a single element), and seq(0.1, 1, by=0.1) for β_3 by using the function expand.grid(). The three vectors of parameter values are collected in a list that is then supplied as the only argument to expand.grid().

```
> grid.Chwirut2 <- expand.grid(list(beta1 = seq(0.1,
+     1, by = 0.1), beta2 = c(0.01),
+     beta3 = seq(0.1, 1, by = 0.1)))
```

The generated grid grid.Chwirut2, which is a data frame, contains three columns with names that correspond to the parameter names, so there is a column for each parameter and as many rows as there are different triples combining elements from the vectors; that is, 100 rows.

In order to evaluate RSS over the grid grid.Chwirut2, the fitting function nls2() in the package of the same name can be used. The specification of nls2() is very similar to that of nls() apart from the start and method arguments. A data frame or even an nls2() model fit can be given as arguments to start. The choice "brute-force" for the argument method evaluates RSS for the parameter values provided through the start argument.

```
> Chwirut2.m2a <- nls2(y ~ expFct(x,
+     beta1, beta2, beta3), data = Chwirut2,
+     start = grid.Chwirut2, algorithm = "brute-force")
```

The resulting output obtained by printing Chwirut2.m2a contains the minimum RSS value and the parameter values for which the minimum was attained.

```
> Chwirut2.m2a

Nonlinear regression model
  model:  y ~ expFct(x, beta1, beta2, beta3)
```

```
data:  NULL
beta1 beta2 beta3
 0.10  0.01  0.10
residual sum-of-squares: 60696
```

```
Number of iterations to convergence: 100
Achieved convergence tolerance: NA
```

The minimum value of RSS attained for the combinations provided in the data frame grid.Chwirut2 is 60696, with corresponding parameter values $(0.1, 0.01, 0.1)$. The obtained nls2() fit Chwirut2.m2a can conveniently be supplied as starting values to nls2() again (not shown). The resulting model fit is similar to the fit Chwirut2.m1 obtained in the previous section.

3.2 Using self-starter functions

We believe that for repeated use of the same nonlinear regression model some automated way of providing starting values is indispensable. The solution is to use self-starter functions.

> Self-starter functions render estimation in nonlinear regression almost as easy and unproblematic as for estimation in linear regression.

Self-starter functions are specific for a given mean function and calculate starting values for a given dataset. Many different self-starter functions can be constructed for a particular mean function. The calculated starting values may not always result in a successful model fit, but robustly designed functions may often yield starting values that are close enough to the parameter estimates that the estimation algorithm will converge.

As pointed out by Watkins and Venables (2006), it is possible to build up knowledge bases within **R**. Once a sensible self-starter function has been constructed for a nonlinear regression model, any future analyses based on this model become considerably easier. We believe that this potential of **R** has not yet been fully realised.

We are only aware of two attempts to create self-starter knowledge bases within **R** designed for use with the fitting function nls(). The primary collection of self-starter functions comes with the standard installation of **R**. We have listed these self-starter functions in Table B.1 in Appendix B. A second collection is found in the package HydroMe and specifically focusses on nonlinear regression models used for estimating soil hydraulic parameters in soil sciences. Finally, a self-starter function for the Richards model is found in the package NRAIA (see Exercise 3.2). In this book, we will only focus on the *built-in* self-starter functions in the standard installation. How to create a self-starter function is the topic of Subsection 3.2.2.

3.2.1 Built-in self-starter functions for nls()

As already mentioned, the function nls() comes with a collection of self-starter functions, which are listed in Table B.1.

L.minor revisited

Let us return to the dataset L.minor. In Section 2.2, a Michaelis-Menten model was fitted to the dataset using nls() with manually supplied starting values. Now we will repeat the model fit using the self-starter function SSmicmen(), which provides a convenient way of fitting the Michaelis-Menten model without having to bother about starting values. We fit the model to L.minor using nls() and SSmicmen(), naming the resulting model fit L.minor.m2.

> *L.minor.m2 <- nls(rate ~ SSmicmen(conc,*
+   *Vm, K), data = L.minor)*

The first argument is again a model formula, where $\sim$ is used to separate the response (rate) on the left-hand side from the self-starter function on the right-hand side. The predictor (conc) is supplied as the first argument in the self-starter function SSmicmen(). The two subsequent arguments in the self-starter function are the two parameters in the mean function, V_m and K, in Equation (2.2) in Subsection 2.2.2. Pay attention to the order of the parameters in the self-starter function (consult for example the relevant help page). The order is determined by the self-starter function; for SSmicmen() it is V_m first and then K. The second argument in nls() is the data frame containing the response and the predictor. When using a self-starter function, there is no need to supply initial parameter values through the argument start. Yet providing the argument start in addition to using a self-starter function will override the starting values found by the self-starter function.

The resulting model fit is identical to the model fit L.minor.m1 that we obtained using manually supplied starting values.

> *summary(L.minor.m2)*

```
Formula: rate ~ SSmicmen(conc, Vm, K)

Parameters:
   Estimate Std. Error t value Pr(>|t|)
Vm  126.033      7.173  17.570 2.18e-06 ***
K    17.079      2.953   5.784  0.00117 **
---
Signif. codes:  0 '***' 0.001 '**' 0.01 '*' 0.05 '.' 0.1 ' ' 1

Residual standard error: 6.25 on 6 degrees of freedom

Number of iterations to convergence: 0
Achieved convergence tolerance: 2.460e-06
```

It is worth noting that the estimation algorithm already converged after the first evaluation, so the number of iterations needed was 0. The reason is that the self-starter function SSmicmen() already employs nls() to find the starting values. This is the case for several of the built-in self-starters.

3.2.2 Defining a self-starter function for nls()

You can make your own self-starter functions. For understanding the following material, it is a prerequisite to know what data frames, functions, lists, and vectors are and how to manipulate them in **R**.

We will illustrate the concept through an example using the exponential model with the mean function

$$f\bigl(x, (b, y_0)\bigr) = y_0 \exp(x/b) \qquad (3.2)$$

This model can be used to describe radioactive decay. The parameter y_0 is the initial amount of the radioactive substance (at time $x = 0$). The rate of decay is governed by the second parameter b (the inverse decay constant).

Apart from the definition of the mean function, the main ingredient in a self-starter function is an initial value routine (Watkins and Venables, 2006), a function taking the dataset as argument as well as a few other arguments that ensures that the initial value routine and the mean function and nls() are tied together and returns starting values ideally not too far from the parameter values. In order to construct such a function, we manipulate Equation (3.2) in such a way that we get a model allowing relatively simple and robust parameter estimation.

Applying a logarithmic transformation on the right-hand side of the exponential model in Equation (3.2) results in the following equation:

$$\log(y_0) + \frac{1}{b}x \qquad (3.3)$$

The relationship between $\log(y)$ and x in Equation (3.3) is linear, with an intercept equal to $\log(y_0)$ and a slope equal to $1/b$. Therefore we can obtain estimates of $\log(y_0)$ and $1/b$ by fitting a linear regression model with $1\log(y)$ as response and x as predictor. We are only interested in getting estimates but do not bother about the error structure, which differs between the original model in Equation (3.2) and the logarithm-transformed model in Equation (3.3) (at most one of them may be the correct one). Therefore the linear regression model should be viewed only as a very crude approximation to the mean function on some transformed scale.

Having boiled down the problem to a linear regression model is convenient because parameter estimation in this model does not involve any iterative procedure. The parameters $\tilde{\beta}_0$ and $\tilde{\beta}_1$ are the estimated intercept and slope, respectively, from the linear regression of $\log(y)$ on x. Initial parameter values of y_0 and b (which we signify using $\sim$ on top) are obtained through back transformation using the exponential and reciprocal functions, respectively:

$$\tilde{y}_0 = \exp(\tilde{\beta}_0), \qquad \tilde{b} = \frac{1}{\tilde{\beta}_1} \tag{3.4}$$

We have now established a procedure for calculating starting values. The next step is to convert the procedure into a corresponding **R** function. We implement the procedure above using the function `selfStart()`, which comes with the standard installation of **R**. Before we use `selfStart()`, we need to define an initial value routine. To this end, we define a function that corresponds to the mean model.

```
> expModel <- function(predictor,
+     b, y0) {
+     y0 * exp(predictor/b)
+ }
```

The function `expModel()` has three arguments. The first argument corresponds to the predictor, whereas the two subsequent arguments are the two parameters in the model, so there is an argument for each parameter (similarly there would need to be one argument for each predictor variable for multivariate predictors). The next step is to define the corresponding initial value routine.

```
> expModelInit <- function(mCall,
+     LHS, data) {
+     xy <- sortedXyData(mCall[["predictor"]],
+         LHS, data)
+     lmFit <- lm(log(xy[, "y"]) ~
+         xy[, "x"])
+     coefs <- coef(lmFit)
+     y0 <- exp(coefs[1])
+     b <- 1/coefs[2]
+     value <- c(b, y0)
+     names(value) <- mCall[c("b",
+         "y0")]
+     value
+ }
```

The arguments supplied to the initial value routine come from within the call that we make to `nls()` when we fit the model. The arguments are as explained below (keep in mind that the initial value routine is invoked from inside `nls()`).

- `mCall`: the `nls()` call where all of the specified arguments are specified by their full names (see the help for `match.call()`)
- `LHS`: the left-hand side in the model formula supplied in the `nls()` call (that is, the response)
- `data`: the data frame used in `nls()`

The following is a line-by-line explanation of the definitions of the initial value routine above:

- *Lines 1–2:* A data frame `xy` with predictor and response values (two columns) sorted according to increasing predictor values is created using the function `sortedXyData()`. The step may be useful as the first step in most initial value routines (for univariate predictors). Note how the name of the first argument in the mean function is referred to as (`"predictor"`); this name needs to correspond exactly to the first argument in the mean function (here `expModel()`).

- *Line 3:* The linear regression model is fit (Equation (3.3)).

- *Line 4:* The parameter estimates are extracted from the fitted linear regression model.

- *Lines 5–6:* The initial value $\tilde{y}_0$ of the parameter y_0 is calculated using the exponential function, and the initial value $\tilde{b}$ of the parameter b is calculated by taking the reciprocal value (using Equation (3.4)).

- *Line 7:* The two initial parameter values are concatenated into a vector named `value`.

- *Line 8:* The components in the vector `value` are given the names specified in the call to the self-starter function, so if, for example, you specify the names `a` and `b`, then those will be the names given to the vector components. This line is needed in order to satisfy the requirement for the argument `start` in `nls()`.

- *Line 9:* Finally, the vector `value` is returned by the initial value routine.

Once the mean function and the initial value routine are defined, the function `selfStart()` can be used to construct the self-starter function:

```
> SSexp <- selfStart(expModel, expModelInit,
+       c("b", "y0"))
```

The third argument specifies the names of the parameters. The self-starter function can be used directly if we want to evaluate the mean function for a given vector of predictor values and given parameter values as in the following example. We use the dataset `RGRcurve` (in the package `nlrwr`), which contains relative growth rates measured over a number of days. The exponential model in Equation (3.2) has been used to fit this dataset (Cedergreen et al., 2005).

```
> with(RGRcurve, SSexp(Day, 4, 0.2))
```

```
[1]  0.2000000 0.2000000 0.2000000
[4]  0.2000000 0.2000000 0.2000000
[7]  0.2568051 0.2568051 0.2568051
[10] 0.2568051 0.2568051 0.3297443
[13] 0.3297443 0.3297443 0.3297443
[16] 0.3297443 0.3297443 0.4234000
[19] 0.4234000 0.4234000 0.4234000
[22] 0.4234000 0.4234000 0.5436564
[25] 0.5436564 0.5436564 0.5436564
[28] 0.5436564 0.5436564 0.8963378
[31] 0.8963378 0.8963378 0.8963378
[34] 0.8963378 0.8963378 1.4778112
[37] 1.4778112 1.4778112 1.4778112
[40] 1.4778112 1.4778112
```

It simply acts as an ordinary mean function, returning values of the mean function for a given data and parameter constellation.

To see the starting values that the self-starter function SSexp() calculates for a specific dataset, the function getInitial() can be used.

```
> getInitial(RGR ~ SSexp(Day, b,
+      y0), data = RGRcurve)

        b         y0
3.8450187 0.1674235
```

Having constructed the self-starter function, the exponential model is conveniently fit as follows.

```
> RGRcurve.m1 <- nls(RGR ~ SSexp(Day,
+      b, y0), data = RGRcurve)
```

The parameter estimates of the model fit RGRcurve.m1 are retrieved using the coef method.

```
> coef(RGRcurve.m1)

        b         y0
3.7645432 0.1637214
```

The starting values obtained from getInitial() above are indeed close to the parameter estimates of the model fit.

More examples on defining self-starter functions for nls() are found in Watkins and Venables (2006) or Venables and Ripley (2002a, pp. 216–217).

Table 3.1. Functions useful for defining self-starter functions.

Name	Usage
getInitial	Calculating the initial values for a given model using a given self-starter function
selfStart	Constructing a self-starter function from a mean function and an initial value routine

Exercises

3.1. The translated generalised hyporbola model defined using the mean function

$$f\big(x, (\theta_1, \theta_2, \theta_3)\big) = \theta_1 + \frac{(\theta_2 - \theta_1)^{\theta_3 + 1}}{(x - \theta_1)^{\theta_3}}$$

has been proposed for these datasets (Hamilton and Knop, 1998). Fit this model to the two datasets btb and sts.

3.2. The Richards growth model is defined using the mean function

$$f\big(x, (b, d, e, f)\big) = d \cdot (1 + \exp((e - x)/b))^{-\exp(-f)}$$

It is a generalisation of the logistic growth model (SSlogis()), which is obtained by setting $f = 0$. Fit the Richards model to the dataset Leaves using the self-starter function SSRichards().

3.3. Construct a self-starter function for nls() for the extended exponential model (encountered in a different guise in Exercise 2.4)

$$f\big(x, (b, c, y_0)\big) = y_0 \exp(x/b) + c$$

which contains a third parameter c representing the lower asymptote or limit that the response approaches for large x values (assuming $b < 0$). Fit the extended exponential model to the dataset wtloss using the constructed self-starter function.

3.4. In Subsection 3.2.2, it is shown how to linearise the mean function of the exponential model. Similarly, the mean function of the Michaelis-Menten model (Equation (2.3)) can be transformed into a linear regression function by using the reciprocal transformation

$$\frac{1}{V_m} + \frac{K}{V_m}\frac{1}{x} = \tilde{\beta}_0 + \tilde{\beta}_1\frac{1}{x}$$

This means that fitting a linear regression model with the response $1/y$ and the predictor $1/x$ will produce estimates of the intercept $\tilde{\beta}_0 = \frac{1}{V_m}$ and the slope

$\tilde{\beta}_1 = \frac{K}{V_m}$. Fit this linear regression model to the dataset L.minor introduced in Subsection 2.2.1. Calculate the derived parameters K and V_m based on the linear regression model fit. Compare the parameter estimates to the summary output given in Subsection 2.2.2.

4

More on nls()

In Chapter 2, we introduced the basic functionality of nls(). In this chapter, we will go into more detail with the arguments and methods available for nls(). We will also provide more examples showing what nls() is capable of.

4.1 Arguments and methods

In Subsection 2.2.2, we specified an nls() call using the following arguments: formula, data, start, and trace. In addition to these arguments, there are several other useful arguments (what follows is not a complete list of arguments, see ?nls all arguments):

- algorithm: specification of estimation algorithm:

  - "default": the Gauss-Newton algorithm (the default)
  - "plinear": for models with conditionally linear parameters (see Section 4.3)
  - "port": for models with constraints on the parameters (can be used with the arguments lower/upper)

- control: fine-tuning of the estimation algorithm (see Section 4.6 for the default values and how to change them)

- na.action: handling of missing values (NAs). The default is na.omit(); other options are na.exclude() and na.fail()

- subset: specification of a subset of the data frame (supplied in the argument data) for which to fit the model

- weights: supplying case weights (see Section 6.4 for an example)

If no starting values are specified for the algorithms "default and "port" (that is, the argument start is not specified), then nls() will use a wild guess: The starting values for all parameters are set to 1. For the "plinear" algorithm, nls() will halt if no starting values are supplied.

Several method functions, or simply methods, are available for extracting specific information from a model fit obtained from nls(). We already used several of them in the previous chapter (e.g., coef and summary). All available methods are listed in Table 4.1. We will use most of these methods in this chapter and subsequent chapters.

Table 4.1. Available methods for extracting various quantities from an nls() model fit.

Name	Usage
anova	comparison of a sequence of nested model fits
coef	parameter estimates from model fit
confint	profile likelihood confidence intervals for the parameters (in the package MASS)
deviance	minimum residual sum of squares $(\mathrm{RSS}(\hat{\beta}))$
df.residual	residual degrees of freedom $(n - p)$
fitted	fitted values: the predictions based on the predictor values in the dataset used
formula	model formula from the model fit
logLik	maximum value of log likelihood value $(\log(L(\hat{\beta}, \hat{\sigma}^2)))$
plot	residual plot (in the package nlme)
predict	predictions based on user-supplied predictor values
print	brief summary output of the model fit
profile	profile t-statistics (see Chapter 7)
residuals	residuals from the model fit
summary	summary output of the model fit
vcov	variance-covariance for the parameter estimates
weights	weights supplied in the nls() call (NULL is returned if no weights were supplied)

We will explain and use many of these methods in this book, but you may still want to consult the help pages for more details.

4.2 Supplying gradient information

Minimisation of RSS using the default Gauss-Newton algorithm relies on a linear approximation of the mean function using the first derivatives of the mean function (that is, gradient information) at each step in the algorithm. If no gradient information is provided, the derivatives are calculated numerically:

nls() uses the function numericDeriv(). Sometimes there may be a benefit in supplying explicit expressions for the derivatives. This may improve the speed of convergence as the number of function evaluations is reduced because such evaluations are used by numericDeriv(), but they are not needed if gradient information is supplied. This could be an issue in situations where a specific model is fitted to many datasets. Continuing with the Michaelis-Menten model and the dataset L.minor from the previous chapters, we show two ways of supplying the gradient information in nls().

4.2.1 Manual supply

Differentiation of the mean function for the Michaelis-Menten model in Equation (2.2) with respect to each of the two parameters K and V_m produces the following partial derivatives:

$$\frac{\partial f}{\partial K} = \frac{-V_m x}{(K+x)^2}$$
$$\frac{\partial f}{\partial V_m} = \frac{x}{K+x} \tag{4.1}$$

Having derived the derivatives available, we can define the enhanced mean function MMfct1() to be supplied to nls(). The function has three arguments: conc, K and Vm (the predictor and the two parameters).

```
> MMfct1 <- function(conc, K, Vm) {
+     numer <- Vm * conc
+     denom <- K + conc
+     mean <- numer/denom
+     partialK <- -numer/(denom^2)
+     partialVm <- mean/Vm
+     attr(mean, "gradient") <- cbind(partialK,
+         partialVm)
+     return(mean)
+ }
```

In the first three lines in the function body between the curly brackets, the mean is calculated and stored in the variable mean. We calculate the numerator, denominator, and their ratio separately because these terms are reused in lines 4–5 in the calculation of the derivatives based on Equation (4.1). In line 6, the vector of calculated mean values defined in line 3 (that is mean) is assigned an attribute, which is a kind of attachment to a variable named gradient and containing the derivatives calculated in lines 4–5. This is the way to attach the gradient information so that nls() will find it. The return value of the function MMfct1() is defined in line 7: The mean values together with the gradient attribute are returned.

The Michaelis-Menten model enhanced with gradient information is fitted to the dataset L.minor as follows.

```
> L.minor.mgr1 <- nls(rate ~ MMfct1(conc,
+    K, Vm), data = L.minor, start = list(K = 20,
+    Vm = 120))
```

The summary output confirms that we obtain a model fit similar to the previous one obtained without using gradient information (the model fit L.minor.m1 from Subsection 2.2.2).

```
> summary(L.minor.mgr1)

Formula: rate ~ MMfct1(conc, K, Vm)

Parameters:
    Estimate Std. Error  t value Pr(>|t|)
K     17.079      2.953    5.784  0.00117 **
Vm   126.033      7.173   17.570 2.18e-06 ***
---
Signif. codes:  0 '***' 0.001 '**' 0.01 '*' 0.05 '.' 0.1 ' ' 1

Residual standard error: 6.25 on 6 degrees of freedom

Number of iterations to convergence: 7
Achieved convergence tolerance: 8.148e-06
```

4.2.2 Automatic supply

The alternative to manually supplying the derivatives is to use the function `deriv()` for deriving symbolic derivatives. This function requires three arguments: the model formula specifying the mean function (the response to the left of the tilde $\sim$ can be skipped, as it is not used), the parameter names, and a function with the predictor and the parameters as arguments and with an empty function body ({ }) to fill in the expressions of the derivatives generated by `deriv()`.

For the Michaelis-Menten model, the call to `deriv()` looks like this:

```
> MMfct2 <- deriv(~Vm * conc/(K +
+    conc), c("K", "Vm"), function(conc,
+    K, Vm) {
+ })
```

The function `MMfct2()` is supplied to `nls()` in the same way as `MMfct1()` in the previous subsection.

```
> L.minor.mgr2 <- nls(rate ~ MMfct2(conc,
+     K, Vm), data = L.minor, start = list(K = 20,
+     Vm = 120))
```

The summary output (not shown) is identical to what we obtained using manual supply.

For a small dataset such as L.minor, there is no benefit in using the gradient information. Venables and Ripley (2002a, pp. 214–216) go through an example involving a larger dataset, where gradient information leads to a reduction in the number of function evaluations. Another example is shown by Fox (2002).

4.3 Conditionally linear parameters

Often the mean function in a nonlinear regression model will not be nonlinear in all parameters. This means the function will be linear in some of the parameters, which we will term conditionally linear parameters (Bates and Watts, 1988, p. 36). Consider again the Michaelis-Menten model:

$$f\bigl(x, (K, V_m)\bigr) = \frac{V_m x}{K + x} \qquad (4.2)$$

This mean function is linear in the parameter V_m. The right-hand side in Equation (4.2) can also be written in the following way by changing the order of the factors:

$$\underbrace{\frac{x}{K + x}}_{\text{coefficient}} \cdot \underbrace{V_m}_{\text{linear term}}$$

The parameter K on the other hand is not conditionally linear, as we cannot establish a similar factorisation of Equation (4.2) for this parameter. Another example is the segmented regression or hockey stick model (Weisberg, 2005, Chapter 11)

$$f\bigl(x, (\theta_0, \theta_1, \gamma)\bigr) = \theta_0 + \theta_1 \max(0, x - \gamma) \qquad (4.3)$$

involving the three parameters θ_0, θ_1, and γ. Here the two parameters θ_0 and θ_1 are conditionally linear.

Parameter estimation can take advantage of conditionally linear parameters because for fixed values of the parameters that are not conditionally linear, the conditionally linear parameters can be estimated using ordinary linear regression. This means that fewer starting values need to be supplied. In the following two subsections we will look at two related ways of exploiting this fact: One approach uses nls() and the other approach uses lm() repeatedly.

4.3.1 nls() using the "plinear" algorithm

To exploit the conditional linear parameters, nls() has to be used with the argument algorithm="plinear". Venables and Ripley (2002a, p. 218) point out that this algorithm may be more robust, not requiring the starting values to be that precise. The model specification is somewhat different from the specification of nls() that we have used so far. For each additive term in the mean function containing a conditionally linear parameter we take what is left after removal of the conditionally linear parameter. This part will only depend on the parameters that are not conditionally linear and the predictor. If there are more additive terms, each of which will correspond to a column, then they need to be bound together subsequently using cbind() (Dalgaard, 2002, Chapter 1) (see Exercise 4.1).

Again, using the L.minor dataset with the Michaelis-Menten model as an example, we find that the model only contains one term: Vm*conc/(K+conc). Omitting the conditionally linear parameter V_m leaves the term conc/(K+conc).

```
> L.minor.m3 <- nls(rate ~ conc/(K +
+    conc), data = L.minor, algorithm = "plinear",
+    start = list(K = 20))
```

The model fit is identical to the model fit L.minor.m1, although the summary output looks slightly different because the conditionally linear parameter is not explicitly named V_m in the nls() call. It is denoted .lin. Note that we only supply a starting value for the parameter K.

```
> summary(L.minor.m3)

Formula: rate ~ conc/(K + conc)

Parameters:
      Estimate Std. Error t value Pr(>|t|)
K       17.079      2.953   5.784  0.00117 **
.lin   126.033      7.173  17.570 2.18e-06 ***
---
Signif. codes:  0 '***' 0.001 '**' 0.01 '*' 0.05 '.' 0.1 ' ' 1

Residual standard error: 6.25 on 6 degrees of freedom

Number of iterations to convergence: 8
Achieved convergence tolerance: 2.058e-06
```

Another example using algorithm="plinear" is found in Venables and Ripley (2002a, pp. 218–220) (here cbind() is used).

4.3.2 A pedestrian approach

In this subsection, we will exploit the conditional linearity in a different way. To this end, the **R** programming needed will become a bit more involved.

Consider the data frame `segreg`. The dataset consists of two variables: C denotes monthly measurements of electricity consumption in kilowatt-hours and Temp is the average temperature in degrees Fahrenheit. Both variables are recorded for one particular building on the University of Minnesota's Twin Cities campus. An initial look at the data in Fig. 4.1 shows that for high temperatures there is an increase in energy consumption as a function of temperature as a consequence of increased use of air conditioning. For low temperatures, energy consumption appears to be constant.

```
> data(segreg)
> plot(C ~ Temp, data = segreg, xlab = Mean ~
+     temperature ~ (degree ~ F),
+     ylab = "Energy consumption (kWh)")
```

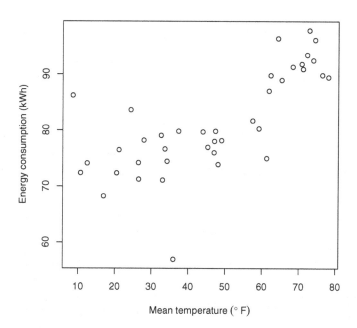

Fig. 4.1. Energy consumption as a function of monthly average temperature based on the data frame `segreg`.

Weisberg (2005, pp. 244–248) considers the segmented regression model defined in Equation (4.3) for the dataset `segreg` (that is, the model with the following mean function):

$$f\big(x, (\theta_0, \theta_1, \gamma)\big) = \theta_0 + \theta_1 \max(0, x - \gamma)$$

Our main interest lies in the parameter γ, which corresponds to the threshold temperature above which increased energy consumption is occurring. As already seen, this parameter is not conditionally linear. Therefore, one option is to consider the profile RSS function for γ, which is a function of γ only because all the remaining parameters are replaced by appropriate estimates. Mathematically, the profile RSS function for γ is defined as follows:

$$\text{RSS}(\gamma) = \min_{\theta_0, \theta_1} \sum_{i=1}^{n} \Big(y_i - f\big(x_i, (\theta_0, \theta_1, \gamma)\big)\Big)^2$$

Thus the value of the profile function for a fixed value of γ is obtained by minimisation of the least squares criterion in the remaining parameters θ_0 and θ_1, so this is a linear regression problem for which `lm()` can be used, as the remaining two parameters are both conditionally linear. Therefore the profile function for the segmented regression model can be defined in **R** as follows:

```
> profRSS1 <- function(gamma) {
+     deviance(lm(C ~ pmax(0, Temp -
+         gamma), data = segreg))
+ }
> profRSS2 <- Vectorize(profRSS1,
+     "gamma")
```

We use the `deviance` method (for `lm()`) to obtain the residual sum-of-square RSS(γ) for a fixed γ value. Then we use the function `Vectorize()` to vectorise the function `profRSS1()` that converts the function from taking a single γ value as argument to taking an entire vector of γ values as argument (automatically doing the calculation for each value in the vector). The first argument to `Vectorize()` is the function to be vectorised (here `profRSS1()`). The second argument is the argument in the function supplied as first argument that should take vector values (here `"gamma"`). The vectorised version of the profile function is useful for plotting the function.

The plot of the profile RSS is shown in Fig. 4.2 based on a crude grid consisting of values of γ corresponding to the actual average temperatures in the dataset (the `Temp` values). The plotted profile function is jagged. This is not only due to the crude grid used but also due to the fact that the mean function is not smooth (it is continuous but not differentiable everywhere). A finer resolution could be achieved by evaluating the profile likelihood function on a finer grid on the temperature axis (see Exercise 4.3), but the bends will remain.

```
> plot(profRSS2(Temp) ~ Temp, data = segreg,
+     type = "l", xlab = expression(gamma),
+     ylab = "Profile RSS")
```

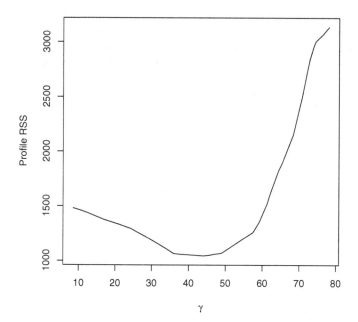

Fig. 4.2. Profile RSS function for the parameter γ for the hockey stick model fitted to the data frame **segreg**. The parameter estimate $\hat{\gamma}$ is lying close to 42.

4.4 Fitting models with several predictor variables

First, we consider an example with two predictors. Second, we show by means of another example how to use nls() for more general models involving several predictors. Our examples only involve two predictors, but they generalise straightforwardly to situations involving more than two predictors.

4.4.1 Two-dimensional predictor

Let us return to the data introduced in Section 1.2. The proposed competition model has the mean function given in Equation (1.5) in Section 1.2, but for convenience we formulate it here again:

$$f\big(x, z, (a, b, c)\big) = \frac{a}{1 + b(x + cz)} \qquad (4.4)$$

The model is fitted to the dataset RScompetition using nls() as follows.

```
> RScompetition.m1 <- nls(biomass ~
+     a/(1 + b * (x + c * z)), data = RScompetition,
+     start = list(a = 20, b = 1,
+         c = 1))
```

So the presence of two predictor variables is not much changing the way
the model is specified. They simply include the mean function specified. The
starting value for a is based on Fig. 1.2. The starting value for b is more
of a guess, whereas the starting value for c has the interpretation that both
biotypes are equally competitive. The summary output is extracted using
summary.

```
> summary(RScompetition.m1)

Formula: biomass ~ a/(1 + b * (x + c * z))

Parameters:
  Estimate Std. Error t value Pr(>|t|)
a  25.9144     2.3393  11.078 1.42e-14 ***
b   0.1776     0.0355   5.004 8.68e-06 ***
c   1.1349     0.2964   3.829 0.000387 ***
---
Signif. codes:  0 '***' 0.001 '**' 0.01 '*' 0.05 '.' 0.1 ' ' 1

Residual standard error: 1.673 on 46 degrees of freedom

Number of iterations to convergence: 8
Achieved convergence tolerance: 1.431e-06
```

The interesting parameter is c, which is estimated to be 1.13. It means that
you need 1.13 resistant plants to substitute for a sensitive plant.

As soon as more than one predictor is considered, it gets difficult to display
the fitted curve together with the original data. There is no general approach,
but for specific models there may be specific solutions providing graphical
displays that succinctly summarise how the model fits the data. For the competition model, such a specific display exists: We can use the term x + cz,
which is often referred to as the virtual or effective density, as the variable on
the horizontal axis and thus reduce the de facto three-dimensional surface imposed by the competition model to a conventional two-dimensional plot. The
calculations necessary in order to plot the biomass as a function of the virtual
density are: (1) to calculate the virtual densities based on the two densities
using the estimate of c, (2) to find the range of the virtual density, and (3) to
calculate the predicted values based on the model fit RScompetition.m1.

```
> virDensity <- with(RScompetition,
+     x + coef(RScompetition.m1)[3] *
+         z)
```

```
> virDenVal <- seq(0, max(virDensity),
+     length.out = 100)
> biomassVal <- predict(RScompetition.m1,
+     data.frame(x = virDenVal, z = 0))
```

The resulting plot is shown in Fig. 4.3, indicating that the model describes the data reasonably well.

```
> plot(biomassVal ~ virDenVal, type = "l",
+     ylab = "Biomass of sensitive biotype (g/plant)",
+     xlab = Virtual ~ density ~
+         (plants/m^2))
> with(RScompetition, points(biomass ~
+     virDensity))
```

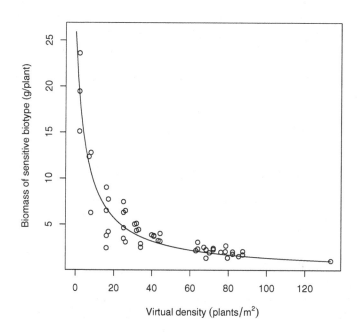

Fig. 4.3. Plot of biomass per plant of the sensitive plants as a function of the virtual density x + 1.13z together with the fitted curve.

4.4.2 General least-squares minimisation

So far, we have used `nls()` for estimating parameters such that the specified mean function fits the data as closely as possible. In other words, we were looking for the parameters minimising the difference $y - f(x, \beta)$ (x and y are playing the roles of predictor and response, respectively) under the least-squares criterion (Equation (2.1)). A more general model formulation is obtained by replacing the difference $y - f(x, \beta)$ by an arbitrary function of the variables x and y, which we want to minimise using the least-squares criterion. If we denote the function to be minimised by, say $\tilde{f}$, then the resulting RSS function looks like this:

$$\text{RSS}(\beta) = \sum_{i=1}^{n} \left(\tilde{f}(x_i, y_i, \beta)\right)^2 \tag{4.5}$$

In this formulation, the variables x and y are partners on equal terms. `nls()` can also be used for least-squares minimisation of arbitrary functions based on Equation (4.5). To demonstrate how this works in practice, we consider an example.

A demodulator is a device that provides a two-dimensional vector representation of an input signal representing the amplitude and phase of the input signal in two components. More background details are provided by Kafadar (1994). The data frame `IQsig` contains such pairs of components from such an input signal (from two channels, named I and Q) measured on an uncalibrated device. The data are shown in Fig. 4.4 using the `plot` method (ignore the superimposed unit circle for the time being).

To ensure a high accuracy in the decomposition carried out by the demodulator, calibration is needed. Kafadar (1994) derives the following implicitly defined nonlinear regression model for the signal values (I_i, Q_i) from an uncalibrated instrument:

$$0 = (I_i - I_0)^2 - 2\gamma \sin(\phi)(I_i - I_0)(Q_i - Q_0) + \gamma^2(Q_i - Q_0)^2 - \left(\rho\gamma\cos(\phi)\right)^2 \tag{4.6}$$

I_0 and Q_0 are the offsets for the I and Q signal values, respectively. γ is the ratio between the amplitudes in the two channels. The angle between the coordinate axes for the I and Q signal values is $\pi/2 - \phi$ radians, and ρ is the amplifier compression ratio. For a perfectly calibrated instrument, the signal (I, Q) would lie on the unit circle in the I/Q coordinate system corresponding to the parameter values: $I_0 = 0$, $\gamma = 1$, $\phi = 0$, $Q_0 = 0$, and $\rho = 1$. This reference unit circle is also shown in Fig. 4.4. It is obtained using the function `lines()`. Figure 4.4 shows that the data deviate from the reference circle by having an elliptical shape, as the circle seems to have become slightly squeezed at the bottom and top.

In order to fit this model, we can specify Equation (4.6) directly in `nls()`, having Equation (4.5) in mind. The left-hand side in the formula supplied to

```
> plot(Q ~ I, data = IQsig)
> theta <- 0:360 * (pi/180)
> lines(cos(theta), sin(theta))
```

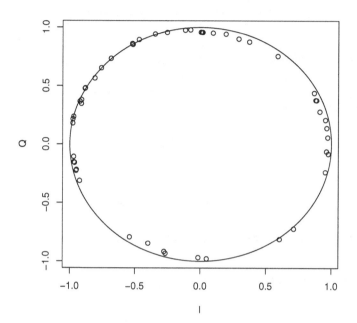

Fig. 4.4. Plot of the original I/Q signal pairs in the dataset **IQsig** together with the reference unit circle corresponding to a perfectly calibrated signal.

nls() is left unspecified, which is interpreted as 0 just like the left-hand side in Equation (4.6). Similarly, the right-hand side in the formula corresponds to the right-hand side in Equation (4.6). The starting values used are close to those suggested in Kafadar (1994). Thus the nls() model specification looks like this:

```
> IQsig.m1 <- nls(~((I - I0)^2 -
+       2 * gamma * sin(phi) * (I -
+           I0) * (Q - Q0) + gamma *
+       gamma * (Q - Q0)^2) - (rho *
+       gamma * cos(phi))^2, data = IQsig,
+       start = list(I0 = -0.005, gamma = 1,
+           phi = -0.005, Q0 = -0.005,
+           rho = 1))
```

The summary output is shown below.

```
> summary(IQsig.m1)

Formula: 0 ~ ((I - I0)^2 - 2 * gamma *
    sin(phi) * (I - I0) * (Q - Q0) +
    gamma * gamma * (Q - Q0)^2) - (rho * gamma * cos(phi))^2

Parameters:
        Estimate Std. Error t value Pr(>|t|)
I0     -0.002259   0.002058  -1.097    0.278
gamma   1.007053   0.003719 270.764  < 2e-16 ***
phi    -0.053540   0.004977 -10.758 5.02e-14 ***
Q0     -0.002481   0.002278  -1.089    0.282
rho     0.974295   0.002540 383.553  < 2e-16 ***
---
Signif. codes:  0 '***' 0.001 '**' 0.01 '*' 0.05 '.' 0.1 ' ' 1

Residual standard error: 0.01917 on 45 degrees of freedom

Number of iterations to convergence: 3
Achieved convergence tolerance: 6.022e-07
```

As could be expected from Fig. 4.4, the estimated offset parameters I_0 and Q_0 are close to (0,0).

4.5 Error messages

Below, we list some of the most common error messages from `nls()`.

The following five error messages usually indicate that the estimation algorithm failed to achieve convergence:

```
Error in nls(... :
  number of iterations exceeded maximum of 50

Error in nls(... :
  step factor 0.000488281 reduced below 'minFactor'
  of 0.000976562

Error in nls(... :
  singular gradient

Error in numericDeriv(form[[3]], names(ind), env) :
  Missing value or an infinity produced when
  evaluating the model
```

```
Error in nlsModel(formula, mf, start, wts) :
  singular gradient matrix at initial parameter estimates
```

The first two messages refer to the fact that the estimation algorithm has reached some *preset limit*:

- The default number of iterations is set to 50. This means that the estimation algorithm will stop after 50 steps regardless of whether or not convergence has been achieved. Sometimes increasing the maximum will help achieve convergence because the procedure simply was terminated prematurely (one example is found in Section 7.6). To see if this is the case, the first thing to do would be to add the argument `trace=TRUE` in the `nls()` specification and rerun `nls()` and then from the trace output assess if the estimates are changing a lot from step to step or are approaching some steady values.

- The step factor is a scaling factor that determines the size of the increment to be added to the estimate from the previous step to obtain the current estimate (this is specific to the Gauss-Newton algorithm). By default, it is set to $1/1024 = 0.0009765625$, but sometimes convergence may be achieved by using a smaller value.

We will explain in the next section how to actually change these default values. The last three error messages are typically related to poor starting values. Solutions could be to:

- choose different starting values (see Chapter 3)
- try another estimation algorithm (the `"port"` algorithm may be more robust than the default Gauss-Newton algorithm)
- reparameterise the mean function (if possible avoiding factors/terms involving several parameters but not involving predictor variables)

Some error messages are related to the use of the self-starter function (occurring before the estimation algorithm gets started). One example is shown below.

```
Error in lm.fit(x, y, offset = offset,
  singular.ok = singular.ok, ...) :
    NA/NaN/Inf in foreign function call (arg 1)
```

For some self-starter functions, such messages may be caused by the presence of 0s among the predictor values. Moreover, the `nls()` fit used in some of the self-starter functions may fail to achieve convergence, and the resulting error messages will then be very similar to the ones listed above. The resulting messages look like this:

```
Error in nls(y ~ cbind(1, 1/(1 + exp((xmid - x)/exp(lscal)))),
  data = xy,    :
```

```
singular gradient
```

```
Error in nls(y ~ 1/(1 + exp((xmid - x)/scal)),
data = xy, start = list(xmid = aux[1],   :
  step factor 0.000488281 reduced below 'minFactor' of
  0.000976562
```

4.6 Controlling nls()

As mentioned in Section 4.1, the fitting function nls() has an argument control for controlling the estimation algorithm. This argument is conveniently specified using the function nls.control(), although it is possible to supply values directly in a list (this is what nls.control() does).

To display the control arguments and their default values, we simply type nls.control() at the command line.

```
> nls.control()

$maxiter
[1] 50

$tol
[1] 1e-05

$minFactor
[1] 0.0009765625

$printEval
[1] FALSE

$warnOnly
[1] FALSE
```

The output is a list with five components.

1. maxiter controls the maximum number of iterations, with a default of 50.
2. tol specifies the tolerance level for the relative offset convergence criterion (Bates and Watts, 1988, pp. 49–50). The closer it is to 0, the more demanding the convergence criterion is. The default is 0.00001.
3. minFactor is the minimum step factor to be used (see the explanation in Section 4.5). The default is $1/1024 = 0.0009765625$.
4. printEval indicates whether or not numerical derivatives should be reported during the estimation for each iteration.
5. warnOnly indicates whether or not nls() should report an error if something goes wrong (e.g., the algorithm fails to converge). If the argument

is set to FALSE (the default), then any error encountered will result in nls() abruptly stopping with an error message. If the argument is set to TRUE, then (for errors producing the first three error messages mentioned in Section 4.5) nls() will issue a warning message and return an *incomplete* model fit instead of stopping with an error. This fit is not appropriate for obtaining parameter estimates and testing hypotheses about the parameters, but it may be useful for finding out what caused the error. It may also be useful to set this argument to TRUE in cases where nls() is used repeatedly for many datasets in an automatic fashion because it prevents the loop through all datasets from stopping due to errors with a few datasets.

More details can be found in the help page ?nls.control.

Exercises

4.1. Fit the hockey stick model to the dataset segreg from Subsection 4.3.2 using the "plinear" algorithm. (Hint: Use the function pmax().) Plot the fitted regression curve together with the data.

4.2. The Deriso stock-recruitment model (Cadima, 2003, p. 48) is defined by

$$f\big(S, (\alpha, c, k)\big) = \alpha S \left(1 - \frac{cS}{k}\right)^{1/c}$$

Fit this model to the dataset M.merluccius. (Hint: It may be an advantage to exploit conditional linearity. Notice also that c is a kind of power parameter, and setting $c = 1$ results in a quadratic regression model with maximum at $S = k$.)

4.3. Consider the analysis of the dataset segreg using the hockey stick model in Subsection 4.3.2. Figure out how to use the function which.min to find the temperature that yields the minimum value of the profile likelihood based on the original temperatures in segreg. Plot the profile likelihood using a finer grid such as tempVal <- seq(35, 50, by = 0.01). Obtain a more precise estimate based on the finer grid.

4.4. Fit the competition model defined in Equation (4.4) to the dataset RScompetition using the following three sets of starting values: $a = 20$, $b = 0$, $c = 1$; $a = 200$, $b = -1$, $c = 100$; and $a = 20$, $b = -1$, $c = 1$. If possible, compare the model fit obtained to the fit found in Subsection 4.4.1.

4.5. The reaction rate of the catalytic isomerisation from n-pentane to isopentane depends on various factors, such as partial pressures of the products involved in the reaction. The data frame Isom contains the partial pressures of hydrogen (H), iso-pentane (I), and n-pentane (N), as well as the corresponding reaction rates. Huet et al. (2004, pp. 9–10) consider the following model for describing the relationship between the reaction rate and the three partial pressures:

$$f\big((H, I, N), (\theta_1, \theta_2, \theta_3)\big) = \frac{\theta_1 \theta_3 (N - I/1.632)}{1 + \theta_2 H + \theta_3 N + \theta_4 I}$$

Fit this nonlinear regression model to the dataset `Isom` (you could again exploit conditional linearity).

5

Model Diagnostics

This chapter is devoted to model checking procedures. Without having validated the assumptions underlying a nonlinear regression model, we cannot be sure that the model is appropriate and consequently that the conclusions based upon the model fit are correct. The kinship to linear regression is apparent, as many of the techniques applicable for linear regression are also useful for nonlinear regression.

If any model violations are found, then Chapter 6 should be consulted.

5.1 Model assumptions

The assumptions underlying nonlinear regression models of the form specified by Equation (1.3) are:

(1) correct mean function f
(2) variance homogeneity (homoscedasticity)
(3) normally distributed measurements errors
(4) mutually independent measurement errors ε_i

Substantive departures from the assumptions could result in bias (inaccurate estimates) and/or distorted standard errors.

Model violations can be detected by means of graphical procedures and formal statistical tests. We believe that graphical procedures will often be sufficient for validating model assumptions, but they may be supplemented by statistical tests. Sometimes, if you are in doubt about the interpretation of a plot, it may be helpful to get a second opinion by using statistical tests. This could be relevant for assessing variance homogeneity and normality assumptions. For nonlinear regression models applied within a regulatory framework (as in toxicity testing), it may indeed be mandatory to carry out such tests (Environment Canada, 2005, pp. 101–103).

In the subsequent four sections, we consider techniques for assessing each of the four assumptions listed above.

5.2 Checking the mean structure

We consider several techniques for assessing the mean structure in nonlinear regression models.

5.2.1 Plot of the fitted regression curve

If the model describes the mean structure in the data appropriately, then the estimated regression curve should agree with the data. Thus we can check the model visually by plotting the data and adding the estimated regression curve. Poor model fits are usually easily spotted. Poor fits may be caused by convergence to suboptimal parameter values that locally (within a smaller region of possible β values), but not globally (among all possible β values) minimise RSS or by choosing a wrong mean model. We will now consider two examples illustrating the latter (have a look at Exercise 4.5 for an illustration of the former).

The first example, which will be the running example in this section and the subsequent sections, is from chemistry and deals with vapour pressure of CO. The dataset vapCO contains measurements of vapour pressure (in Pa) of carbon monoxide (CO) for a range of different temperatures (in K). The dataset is shown in Fig. 5.1.

Based on theoretical considerations, the Clapeyron model has been derived. It relates the logarithm-transformed pressure to temperature through the following equation:

$$\log(\text{pressure}) \approx A - \frac{B}{\text{temperature}} \tag{5.1}$$

This is an ordinary linear regression model (predictor: $\frac{1}{\text{temperature}}$, intercept: A, slope: B) providing a rough approximation to the relationship between pressure and temperature. An empirically based modification of the Clapeyron model in Equation (5.1) that provides an improved description of the relationship is the three-parameter Antoine model (Van Ness and Abbott, 1997, pp. 4–15) given by the relationship

$$\log(\text{pressure}) \approx A - \frac{B}{C + \text{temperature}} \tag{5.2}$$

with the additional parameter being denoted C. The Antoine model is a nonlinear regression model with mean function

$$f(\text{temperature}, (A, B, C)) = A - \frac{B}{C + \text{temperature}}$$

We fit the Antoine model in Equation (5.2) to the dataset vapCO using nls() (notice that the response is logarithm-transformed (log(p))).

```
> plot(p ~ T, data = vapCO, log = "y",
+     xlab = "Temperature (K)", ylab = "Pressure (Pa)")
```

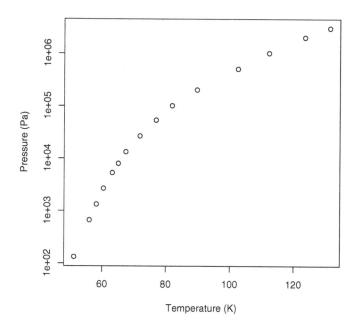

Fig. 5.1. Plot of the dataset vapCO showing the relationship between pressure and temperature for CO. Notice that the pressure axis is logarithmic as in Equation (5.1).

```
> vapCO.m1 <- nls(log(p) ~ A - B/(C +
+     T), data = vapCO, start = list(A = 10,
+     B = 100, C = -10))
```

The response used is the logarithm-transformed pressure. The plot of the data together with the estimated regression curve is shown in Fig. 5.2.

Notice that we are back-transforming the fitted values from the logarithm axis using the exponential function exp(). We see that there is quite good agreement between the original data and the estimated regression curve, indicating that the model is capturing the systematic part in the data appropriately.

The second example uses the dataset lettuce in the package drc, which is the result of a typical dose-response experiment, where lettuce plant biomass is expected to decrease as the concentration of the chemical isobutyl alcohol is increased, and eventually the plant is killed, resulting in a plant biomass close to 0 (van Ewijk and Hoekstra, 1993). Seven isobutyl alcohol concentrations

```
> plot(p ~ T, data = vapCO, log = "y",
+       xlab = "Temperature (K)", ylab = "Pressure (Pa)")
> lines(vapCO$T, exp(fitted(vapCO.m1)))
```

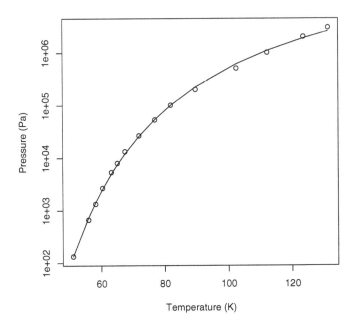

Fig. 5.2. Plot of the dataset `vapCO` together with the estimated regression curve based on the Antoine model.

were used, with two replicates per concentration, amounting to a dataset of size 14.

For such a toxicity experiment, it is common to use the log-logistic model with a lower limit fixed at 0 (van Ewijk and Hoekstra, 1993). The corresponding mean function is defined as follows:

$$f\big(x, (b, d, e)\big) = \frac{d}{1 + \left(\frac{x}{e}\right)^b} \tag{5.3}$$

This model corresponds to a strictly decreasing dose-response curve, but looking at Fig. 5.3, it is apparent that such a curve will not describe the nonmonotonous pattern in the data well. Therefore a nonmonotonous mean function is required to describe this type of data. The phenomenon seen in Fig. 5.3 is often called hormesis. Such models are discussed by Brain and Cousens (1989), Cedergreen et al. (2005), and Beckon et al. (2008).

```
> plot(weight ~ conc, data = lettuce,
+     xlab = "Concentration (mg/l)",
+     ylab = "Biomass (g)", log = "x")
```

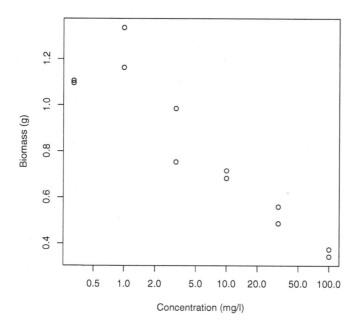

Fig. 5.3. Plot of biomass as a function of concentration for the dataset `lettuce` (using a logarithmic concentration axis).

Plotting the data and the estimated regression curve is only really useful for one-dimensional predictors. For multidimensional predictors, we will have to use other approaches, such as the one introduced in the next subsection.

5.2.2 Residual plots

In Subsection 5.2.1, the appropriateness of the model fit was inspected by assessing whether or not the data were spread in a nonsystematic/random manner around the fitted nonlinear regression curve (Fig. 5.2). Often it is easier to look for deviations from a horizontal line. This can be accomplished using residual plots. The raw or working residual $\hat{r}_i$ for the ith observation is the part of the response value that is not captured by the model. More precisely, the residual is defined as the difference between the response value y_i and the corresponding fitted value:

$$\hat{r}_i = y_i - f(x_i, \hat{\beta}) \qquad (5.4)$$

The residual plot is the plot of the fitted values (defined in Subsection 2.2.3) versus the residuals (plotting the pairs $(f(x_i, \hat{\beta}), \hat{r}_i)$). It is worth noting that the residual plot is also well-defined for multivariate predictors, even though in this situation it could also be relevant to plot the residuals against each component of the predictor.

When looking at the residual plot, you should keep the following question in mind: Is there any systematic pattern in the plot? If yes, then the mean function is not appropriate for describing the data at hand. If no, then the mean function is adequately capturing the average trend in the data. Clearly, there is a grey zone where it can be difficult to decide. A systematic pattern may often manifest itself in the form of curvature or trends in the plot, for instance rendering the plot asymmetric around the x axis. This indicates that the mean function is not doing a good job of describing the average behaviour of data.

We saw already in Subsection 2.2.3 how to obtain the fitted values. The residuals are retrieved from the `nls()` model fit by applying the `residuals` method. The residual plot for the model fit `vapCO.m1` obtained in Subsection 5.2.1 is shown in Fig. 5.4. The points in Fig. 5.4 correspond to pairs of fitted values and residuals: There seems to be some curvature in the plot, as the residuals fluctuate from groups of negative residuals to groups of positive residuals and then back again, so maybe the Antoine model is not describing the data in `vapCO` that well after all.

5.2.3 Lack-of-fit tests

If there are replicates available (that is, repeated measurements at the same value of x), then it is possible to supplement the graphical assessment of the mean function with statistical tests.

The idea is to compare the chosen nonlinear regression model to a more general ANOVA model. We consider the dataset `ryegrass` in the package `drc`. The data are from a study investigating the joint action of phenolic acid mixtures on root growth inhibition of perennial ryegrass (*Lolium perenne L.*) and its significance in allelopathy research (Inderjit et al., 2002). The toxicity of ferulic acid (one component in the mixtures mentioned before) when applied to perennial ryegrass was examined for a range of concentrations. The response is the root length of perennial ryegrass plants in cm (`rootl`), and the predictor is the concentration of ferulic acid in mM (`conc`). Figure 5.5 shows the data.

It was established in Inderjit et al. (2002) that the four-parameter log-logistic model is appropriate for describing the decline in growth caused by ferulic acid.

$$f\big(x, (b, c, d, e)\big) = c + \frac{d - c}{1 + \left(\frac{x}{e}\right)^b} \qquad (5.5)$$

```
> plot(fitted(vapCO.m1), residuals(vapCO.m1),
+    xlab = "Fitted Values", ylab = "Residuals")
> abline(a = 0, b = 0)
```

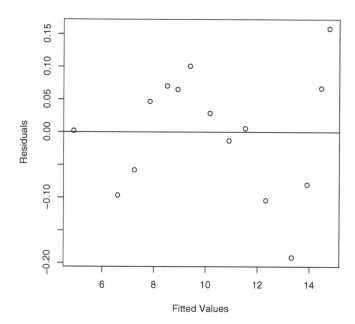

Fig. 5.4. Residual plot based on the model fit vapCO.m1 of the Antoine model fitted to the dataset vapCO. A reference line with intercept 0 and slope 0 has been added using abline().

This is the model that we introduced in Section 1.3. If we were to ignore all the biological knowledge above on how the response, root length, is expected to depend on the predictor, herbicide concentration, we could choose to analyse the dataset using a one-way ANOVA model with conc as a factor (Dalgaard, 2002, pp. 111–120). The one-way ANOVA model imposes no restrictions on how the response changes from one concentration to another concentration, as there will be one parameter for each concentration. Consequently, it is a more general model than the nonlinear regression model, or, in other words, the nonlinear regression model is a submodel of the ANOVA model. This means that we can compare the ANOVA model and the nonlinear regression model using a statistical test, testing the null hypothesis that the ANOVA model can be simplified to the nonlinear regression model. This test is called the lack-of-fit test. We consider two approaches for testing the hypothesis:

- the F-test (Bates and Watts, 1988, pp. 103–104)

```
> plot(rootl ~ conc, data = ryegrass,
+     xlab = "Concentration (mM)",
+     ylab = "Root length (cm)")
```

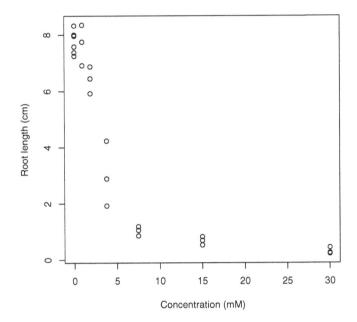

Fig. 5.5. Plot of the root length for a range of concentrations of ferulic acid using the dataset **ryegrass**.

- the likelihood ratio test (Huet et al., 2004, pp. 110–111)

F-test

The F-test statistic is a measure of the distance between the ANOVA model and nonlinear model expressed as the difference of the sums-of-squares terms for the two models relative to the size of the sums-of-squares term for the more general model. A large value of the statistic indicates that the two models are far apart, meaning that they do not provide similar descriptions of the data, and consequently the more general ANOVA model is the more appropriate model.

A brief definition of the F-test statistic is that it is a ratio with the numerator being the difference in the sums-of-squares terms between the two models being compared divided by the difference in parameters between the two models and the denominator being the sums-of-squares term for the more general of the two models, the ANOVA model. The F-test statistic is defined as follows:

$$F = \frac{(\text{RSS}(\hat{\beta}) - \text{RSS}_{\text{ANOVA}})/(n - p - df_{\text{ANOVA}})}{\text{RSS}_{\text{ANOVA}}/df_{\text{ANOVA}}}$$

The F-test statistic is defined in exactly the same way as for linear models, but in contrast to linear models the F-distribution only holds approximately (getting better as the sample size increases). The p-value is determined by looking up the value of the F-statistic in an F-distribution with degrees of freedom $(n - p - df_{\text{ANOVA}}, df_{\text{ANOVA}})$, where df_{ANOVA} denotes the degrees of freedom in the ANOVA model (the number of observations minus the number of distinct predictor values).

If there are no replicates for any of the predictor values in the dataset, then the term $\text{RSS}_{\text{ANOVA}}$ is 0 and the test is not defined.

What can we conclude from the test? If the test is nonsignificant (e.g., using a significance level of 0.05), then there is no evidence against the non-linear regression model. If the test is significant, however, then the nonlinear regression model may not be appropriate. We are purposely cautious in formulating the interpretation of the lack-of-fit test, as the test is sensitive to the variation in data: A small variation may result in a significant test even though the model seems appropriate (e.g., the model fitted similar data in the past with no problems), whereas a large variation may yield a nonsignificant and inconclusive result.

To obtain the F-test for a model fitted with nls(), we first need to fit the more general ANOVA model. This is accomplished using the function lm for fitting linear models (Dalgaard, 2002, Chapter 5).

```
> ryegrass.m1 <- lm(rootl ~ as.factor(conc),
+      data = ryegrass)
```

Notice that we convert the variable conc to a factor (Dalgaard, 2002, pp. 111–120) in order to fit a one-way ANOVA model. Next we fit the log-logistic model using nls().

```
> ryegrass.m2 <- nls(rootl ~ c +
+      (d - c)/(1 + exp(b * +(log(conc) -
+          log(e)))), start = list(b = 1,
+      c = 0.6, d = 8, e = 3), data = ryegrass)
```

The lack-of-fit test is then obtained using anova with two arguments: the nonlinear regression fit as the first argument and the ANOVA fit as the second argument.

```
> anova(ryegrass.m2, ryegrass.m1)
```

Analysis of Variance Table

```
Model 1: rootl ~ c + (d - c)/(1 + exp(b * +(log(conc) - log(e))))
Model 2: rootl ~ as.factor(conc)
  Res.Df Res.Sum Sq Df Sum Sq F value
1   20      5.4002
2   17      5.1799  3 0.2204  0.2411
  Pr(>F)
1
2 0.8665
```

The lack-of-fit test is overwhelmingly nonsignificant, which lends support to the nonlinear regression model. We conclude that the four-parameter log-logistic model is appropriate for describing the relation between the response and the predictor in the dataset ryegrass.

Likelihood ratio test

An alternative to the F-test is to use a lack-of-fit test based on a likelihood ratio test. Like the F-test, the likelihood ratio test is a test for comparison of two nested models, where one model is more general than the other model. The test statistic itself is defined as -2 times the difference of the logarithms of the likelihood functions for the nonlinear regression model (Subsection 2.2.2) and the ANOVA model (evaluated at the optimal parameter value). The resulting test statistic Q is given by the expression

$$Q = n \log \mathrm{RSS}(\hat{\beta}) - n \log \mathrm{RSS}_{\mathrm{ANOVA}}$$

Large values of Q lead to rejection of the nonlinear regression model. To determine what a large value is, we assume that Q is approximately χ^2-distributed with $n - p - df_{\mathrm{ANOVA}}$ degrees of freedom.

The lack-of-fit test is obtained with the logLik method applied to the two model fits ryegrass.m1 and ryegrass.m2 and then taking -2 times their difference (the submodel coming first in the difference).

```
> Q <- -2 * (logLik(ryegrass.m2) -
+    logLik(ryegrass.m1))
```

The corresponding degrees of freedom is obtained using the df.residual method.

```
> df.Q <- df.residual(ryegrass.m2) -
+    df.residual(ryegrass.m1)
```

Finally, the p-value of the lack-of-fit test based on a likelihood ratio test is obtained by evaluating Q in the χ^2 distribution with df.Q degrees of freedom using the cumulative distribution function pchisq().

```
> 1 - pchisq(Q, df.Q)
```

```
'log Lik.' 0.8012878 (df=5)
```

We find that the p-value is not far from the p-value of the F-test.

5.3 Variance homogeneity

In this section, we will focus on assumption (2) in Section 5.1 using the dataset vapCO.

5.3.1 Absolute residuals

Variance inhomogeneity can be detected by looking at a plot of the fitted values versus the absolute residuals , which are defined as follows:

$$|\hat{r}_i| = \begin{cases} \hat{r}_i & \hat{r}_i \geq 0 \\ -\hat{r}_i & \hat{r}_i < 0 \end{cases}$$

The absolute residuals are the raw residuals stripped for negative signs. Again we can use plot in combination with the fitted and residuals methods and the function abs() for obtaining absolute values. The resulting plot is shown is Fig. 5.6.

In Fig. 5.6, there seems to be an overall, though somewhat jagged, increasing trend with increasing fitted values. We would say that the variance is an increasing function of the mean. This indicates that the assumption of variance homogeneity is not satisfied. In Chapter 6, we will discuss how to remedy this type of model violation.

5.3.2 Levene's test

If there are replicates available, then the graphical procedure in the previous subsection can be supplemented by means of a statistical test.

A robust test for examining the hypothesis of equal variances at all predictor values is Levene's test (Environment Canada, 2005). The test is robust in the sense that it does not rely on the normality assumption. In **R**, this test is available in the package car (which was loaded together with nlrwr) through the function levene.test().

```
> with(ryegrass, levene.test(root1,
+     as.factor(conc)))

Levene's Test for Homogeneity of Variance
      Df F value Pr(>F)
group  6  1.9266 0.1344
      17
```

The test indicates that the assumption of variance homogeneity is satisfied. A nonrobust alternative is Bartlett's test, available in **R** through the function bartlett.test().

```
> plot(fitted(vapCO.m1), abs(residuals(vapCO.m1))),
+     xlab = "Fitted values", ylab = "Absolute residuals")
```

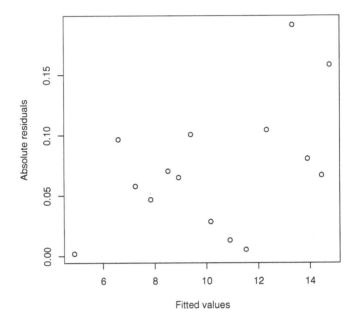

Fig. 5.6. Plot of the absolute residuals for the model fit `vapCO.m1` of the Antoine model to the dataset `vapCO`.

5.4 Normal distribution

The distribution of the measurement errors may deviate from the normality assumption in many ways. A few possibilities are one or few outliers, too many extreme values (heavy tails), or skewness. Such deviations can be assessed using the standardised residuals (Pinheiro and Bates, 2000, pp. 149–150), which are defined as the raw residuals divided by the square root of the estimated residual variance:

$$\hat{e}_i = \hat{r}_i/s$$

If the model assumptions are satisfied, then the standardised residuals will be approximately standard normally distributed (having expectation 0 and deviation 1). They are not entirely independent, but usually the correlation is small. Therefore the plot of the fitted values versus the standardised residuals, obtained using the **plot** method, can be useful in assessing whether or not the spread of the standardised residuals resembles that of a standard normal distribution. There are several arguments that can be specified for the plot method and are useful for identifying observations; see the help page ?plot.nls for more details. The resulting plot for the model fit vapCO.m1 is shown in Fig. 5.7. Note that, apart from the scale on the y axis, the plot looks very much like the one in Fig. 5.4.

```
> plot(vapCO.m1)
```

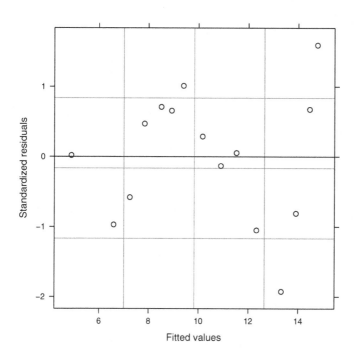

Fig. 5.7. Plot of the fitted values versus the standardised residuals for the nls() model fit vapCO.m1.

The plot of the fitted values versus the standardised residuals may be of some help in detecting deviations from the normal distribution (such as heavy-tailed distributions or outliers). However, it is often more informative to look at the standardised residuals in a QQ plot.

5.4.1 QQ plot

A normal QQ plot compares the distribution of the standardised residuals to a standard normal distribution (see Dalgaard, 2002, p. 64). The two distributions agree if the points in the QQ plot approximately follow a straight line intercepting the y axis at 0 and having slope 1. The QQ plot can be made by qqnorm(). The QQ plot for the nonlinear regression fit ryegrass.m2 is shown in Fig. 5.8. We use abline() to add the reference line. The standardised residuals are obtained using the residual method and then subsequently dividing by the estimated residual error, which is extracted as the component "sigma" for the summary output of the model fit.

```
> standardRes <- residuals(ryegrass.m2)/summary(ryegrass.m2)$sigma
> qqnorm(standardRes, main = "")
> abline(a = 0, b = 1)
```

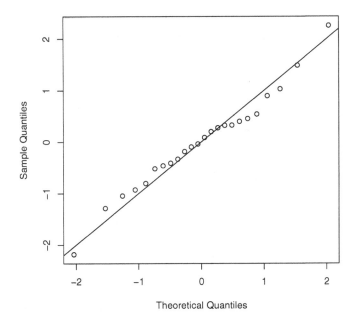

Fig. 5.8. Normal QQ plot for the model fit ryegrass.m2 of the log-logistic model to the dataset ryegrass. The reference line with intercept 0 and slope 1 is also shown.

Taking the small number of observations into account, the QQ plot shows good agreement between the two distributions, and we have reason to believe that the normality assumption is satisfied. In some situations (especially for small datasets), it may be useful to have a statistical test as an aid for deciding whether or not the normality assumption is met. The next subsection introduces such a test.

5.4.2 Shapiro-Wilk test

The Shapiro-Wilk test can be used to assess whether or not the residuals are normally distributed. This test is available within the standard installation of R through the function shapiro.test, which takes the vector for residuals from the model fit as its argument. So, for the model fit ryegrass.m2, the Shapiro-Wilk test is obtained as follows (we reuse the vector standardRes of standardised residuals constructed above).

```
> shapiro.test(standardRes)

    Shapiro-Wilk normality test

data:  standardRes
W = 0.9823, p-value = 0.9345
```

We see that the test confirms the visual impression from the QQ plot in Fig. 5.8: The assumption of normally distributed errors is acceptable. The value of the test statistic (the closer to 1, the better the agreement in Fig. 5.8) and the resulting p-value should not be given too much weight. Use it as supplement to the QQ plot.

5.5 Independence

Typically, for designed experiments such as the one leading to the dataset ryegrass used in Subsection 5.2.3, independence between response values is ensured by the experimental design using a new organism or subject for each measurement. Correlated response values often occur in experiments where repeated measurements on the same organism or subject occur. A few examples are:

- all measurements stem from the same organism or subject
- replicate measurements at each predictor value are from the same organism or subject

Ignoring correlation will tend to give the wrong precision of parameter estimates. Sometimes arguments specific to the subject matter can rule out correlation; see Ducharme and Fontez (2004) for an example of biological reasoning related to modelling growth curves.

One way to detect correlation is to look at a *lag plot*, which is a plot of each raw residual versus the previous residual (also called the lag-one residual) in the order determined by the predictor scale. Correlation would show up as a linear trend; examples are given by Bates and Watts (1988, pp. 92–96) and Huet et al. (2004, p. 106).

For the model fit vapCO.m1, the lag plot is shown in Fig. 5.9 below. We obtain the lagged residuals using residuals(vapCO.m1)[-1], simply taking the vector of residuals and leaving out the first component. To match the lengths of the vectors, we append an NA to the vector of lagged residuals. There appears to be a positive linear relationship in the plot. However, there is quite some scatter in the plot, and therefore we cannot be very certain about this trend.

```
> plot(residuals(vapCO.m1), c(residuals(vapCO.m1)[-1],
+    NA), xlab = "Residuals", ylab = "Lagged residuals")
```

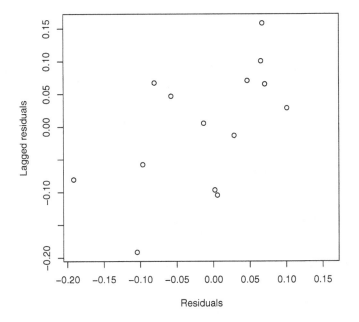

Fig. 5.9. Lag plot of the model fit vapCO.m1 for the Antoine model fitted to the dataset vapCO.

Exercises

5.1. Fit the Clapeyron model to the dataset vapCO. Carry out model checking.

5.2. A classical model for population growth is the logistic or Verhulst model, which describes the population size through the mean function

$$f\big(\text{time}, (\beta_1, \beta_2, \beta_3)\big) = \frac{\beta_1}{1 + \exp(\beta_2 + \beta_3\text{time})}$$

β_1 is the upper limit for population growth, β_2 is related to the population size at time 0 (the population size is not 0 at time 0), and β_3 (< 0) governs the rate of growth. The dataset US.pop contains the population size of the United States of America from 1790 to 1990 (per decade). Plot population size versus decades. Fit the logistic model. Check the model assumptions (what is your conclusion?).

5.3. Make a plot of the dataset heartrate. Fit a log-logistic model (Equation (5.5)) to the dataset. Check the model assumptions.

5.4. The reason for the poor fit obtained for the dataset lettuce in Subsection 5.2.1 is that there appears to be a hormetic effect at low concentrations, an initial stimulation contrary to the expected effect of the herbicide. Only at higher concentrations is the expected effect of the herbicide visible. The Brain-Cousens model

$$f\big(x, (b, d, e, f)\big) = \frac{d + f \cdot x}{1 + (x/e)^b}$$

is specifically intended for describing hormesis. Fit this model to the dataset lettuce. Check the model assumptions.

5.5. Consider the nonlinear regression model fit

```
> Indometh.1.m1 <- nls(conc ~ SSbiexp(time,
+     A1, lrc1, A2, lrc2), data = Indometh,
+     subset = Subject == 1)
```

which is fitted to a subset of the dataset Indometh (see ?Indometh for a detailed description). Check the model assumptions. Are there any substantive deviations?

6

Remedies for Model Violations

In the previous chapters, we assumed that the measurement errors were standard normally distributed (with mean 0 and variance σ^2). In this chapter, we consider several approaches for dealing with model violations related to the measurement errors:

- normally distributed with heterogeneous variance
- non-normally distributed with homogeneous or heterogeneous variance

Modelling the variance will only remove variance heterogeneity, but it is no remedy for non-normal errors. In contrast, a transformation approach may often be able to remediate both non-normal error distributions and variance heterogeneity.

6.1 Variance modelling

Variance heterogeneity usually will not influence the parameter estimates $\hat{\beta}$ much, but if ignored it may result in severely misleading confidence and prediction intervals (Carroll and Ruppert, 1988, pp. 51–61).

One way of taking into account variance heterogeneity is by explicitly modelling it; that is, formulating a regression model for the variance similar to what we have done for the mean in Equation (1.3). Thus we will assume that the mean is specified as in Equation (1.3) and, furthermore, that the errors are additive and normally distributed.

In Chapter 2, we assumed that all errors had the same variance,

$$\text{var}(\varepsilon_i) = \sigma^2 \tag{6.1}$$

implying that the errors were identically distributed. Now we will consider situations where the variance changes as the predictor values change.

6.1.1 Power-of-the-mean variance model

Often the variance is nonconstant in such a way that it depends on the mean: A small mean value implies a small variance, whereas a large mean value implies a large variance (it can also be the other way around). Consider the plot in Fig. 6.1, which shows exponential growth of relative growth rates as a function of time based on the dataset RGRcurve already used in Subsection 3.2.2. There is a clear tendency: the larger the mean value, the larger the variation around the mean value.

```
> plot(RGR ~ Day, data = RGRcurve,
+    xlab = "Time (days)", ylab = "Relative growth rate (%)")
```

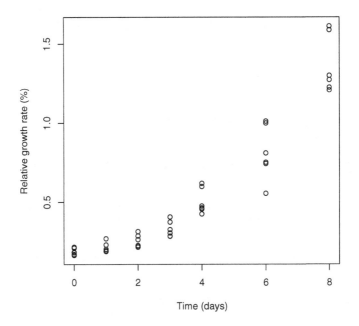

Fig. 6.1. Relative growth rate as a function of time in days.

One way to model the dependence of the variance on the mean seen in Fig. 6.1 is through a power-of-the-mean variance model

$$\text{var}(\varepsilon_i) = \sigma^2 \big(f(x_i, \beta) \big)^{2\theta} \qquad (6.2)$$

where the variance of each observation y_i depends on the corresponding mean value $f(x_i, \beta)$ through a power function with exponent 2θ. Variance homogeneity corresponds to $\theta = 0$, in which case Equation (6.2) reduces to Equation (6.1). This means that the model with variance homogeneity is a submodel of the power-of-the-mean model and, consequently, a statistical test can be used to assess whether or not the power-of-the-mean model provides a significantly improved fit compared with the model that assumes variance homogeneity.

The parameter θ is usually assumed to be unknown and will have to be estimated from data, though in some situations the data type would justify fixing θ at a certain value. If the response values are counts that are not too small then they may be treated as if they are normally distributed with a variance structure mimicking that of the Poisson distribution: $\text{var}(\varepsilon_i) = \sigma^2 f(x_i, \beta)$ ($\theta = 1/2$) (see Huet et al., 2004, pp. 222–224).

For estimation of the regression parameters as well as the variance parameter θ, several approaches are available. In **R**, the function gnls() in the package nlme allows generalised least squares estimation of the power-of-the-mean model (Equation (6.2)) and a few related built-in variance models (see Table 6.1 below). The details behind the estimation procedure implemented in gnls() are found in Pinheiro and Bates (2000, pp. 332–336).

Returning to the dataset RGRcurve, we want to fit an exponential growth model (Equation (3.2)). We use gnls(), which is specified in much the same way as nls(). We use the self-starter defined in Subsection 3.2.2.

```
> RGRcurve.m2 <- gnls(RGR ~ SSexp(Day,
+       a, b), data = RGRcurve, weights = varPower())
```

Apart from the last argument, the specified arguments are the same as for an nls() call: first the model formula using the previously defined self-starter function (Subsection 3.2.2), then the dataset containing the variables used in the formula. The last argument, weights, specifies the variance model varPower(), where the variance is a power of a predictor or the mean. The default is a power-of-the-mean variance model. The default argument in full in varPower() looks like

```
weights = varPower( form =  fitted(.) )
```

which means that the variance is a power of the fitted values. For more details, consult Pinheiro and Bates (2000, pp. 401–409). If the argument weights is omitted, gnls() produces the same model fit as nls(). The summary method (as well as most other standard methods) is available for models fitted with gnls().

```
> summary(RGRcurve.m2)

Generalized nonlinear least squares fit
  Model: RGR ~ SSexp(Day, a, b)
  Data: RGRcurve
       AIC       BIC    logLik
  -97.20773 -90.35344 52.60386

Variance function:
 Structure: Power of variance covariate
 Formula: ~fitted(.)
 Parameter estimates:
  power
1.012692

Coefficients:
     Value  Std.Error  t-value p-value
a 3.858027 0.14751689 26.15312       0
b 0.168432 0.00720728 23.36973       0

 Correlation:
  a
b 0.797

Standardized residuals:
      Min         Q1        Med
-1.8325511 -0.6356797 -0.1609886
       Q3        Max
0.6477644  1.8176431

Residual standard error: 0.1671879
Degrees of freedom: 41 total; 39 residual
```

The summary output consists of the following six components: (1) model specification and measures of goodness-of-fit, (2) estimated variance parameters, (3) estimated parameters in the mean model, (4) estimated correlation between parameters in the mean model, (5) five-number summary of the distribution of the residuals, and (6) estimated residual standard error. Below we provide an explanation for each component.

(1) First, the specified model formula is shown. Second, the name of the data frame used is listed. Third, the values of the goodness-of-fit measures AIC (Akaike's information criterion), BIC (Bayesian information criterion), and the logarithm of the likelihood function are displayed. The AIC and BIC are useful for comparing models that are non-nested (Burnham and Anderson, 2002, Chapter 2), but at the moment we only

consider a single model and therefore have no use for these measures (see Section 7.6 for an example of how to use these measures). The value of the log likelihood function can be used to compare nested models through a likelihood ratio test using a χ^2 distribution as reference (see Subsection 5.2.3 for an example).

(2) The variance structure used and the estimated variance parameter are displayed. The variance parameter estimate $\hat{\theta}$ is 1.01, really close to 1, indicating that the variance structure resembles that of a gamma distribution (Nelder, 1991); that is, the variance is proportional to the square of the mean.

(3) This part of the output is similar to the output from an nls() model, showing the parameter estimates with the corresponding standard errors and t-test statistic and p-value for the null hypothesis that the parameter is equal to 0. The parameter estimates have not changed much compared with the model fit that assumes constant variance (RGRcurve.m1 in Subsection 3.2.2).

(4) The estimated correlation between the parameter estimates is reported. In our example, it is a single number, as we consider a mean function with only two parameters). The estimates of the parameters in the mean function will be mutually correlated to a lesser or greater extent.

(5) The five-number summary consists of the minimum, maximum, median, and 25% and 75% quantiles of the distribution of the standardised residuals. This summary may be useful for assessing whether the standardised residuals are evenly spread around 0 (looking at the summary, we find that the median is close to 0, and the 25% and 75% quantiles are similar apart from the sign; the minimum and maximum are also similar apart from the sign).

(6) The residual standard error is 0.167, and the residual degrees of freedom is 39, obtained as the difference between 41 (number of observations) and 2 (number of parameters).

The self-starter functions that are available for nls() also work for gnls(). Other examples using gnls() in conjunction with varPower are found in the help page of gnls() (?gnls) and in Pinheiro and Bates (2000, pp. 401–404).

6.1.2 Other variance models

Apart from the power-of-the-mean model (varPower()), a few other variance models can be specified. The most important models are listed in Table 6.1 below.

The package nlreg in the bundle hoa also provides functionality for fitting nonlinear regression models that assume various variance structures (Brazzale, 2005).

Table **6.1.** Variance models for use with `gnls()`.

R function	Variance model
`varExp()`	Variance as exponential of covariate or mean
`varIdent()`	Different variances in different groups
`varPower()`	Variance as power of covariate or mean

6.2 Transformations

Frequently the response values are both non-normally distributed and exhibit variance heterogeneity. For example, right-skewed response values (e.g., lengths or weights of some test organisms) with variation that increases as a function of the mean are commonly encountered in toxicology (OECD (Organisation for Economic Cooperation and Development), 2006a). In such situations, it may often be possible to find a transformation that will produce nearly normally distributed response values with constant variance. This approach for nonlinear regression was introduced by Carroll and Ruppert (1984) and elaborated in Carroll and Ruppert (1988, Chapter 4). It has also been discussed by Streibig et al. (1993) in a weed science context.

6.2.1 Transform-both-sides approach

In Section 1.1, we encountered a model that is used in fisheries management, namely the Beverton-Holt model. For modelling the stock-recruitment relationship between sockeye salmon in the Skeena River, Carroll and Ruppert (1988, pp. 139–152) consider another two-parameter nonlinear regression model for the relationship between stock (S) and recruitment (number of recruits):

$$f\big(S, (\alpha, k)\big) = \alpha S \exp(-kS) \qquad (6.3)$$

This model is called the Ricker model, and it was derived from theoretical considerations. As in the Beverton-Holt model, the parameter α has the same interpretation as the slope of the tangent at 0. The mean function in Equation (6.3) tends to 0 both for S approaching 0 from the right and for S approaching ∞, and it has a maximum at $S = 1/k$, so this mean function is not monotonous in S.

The data are provided in the data frame `sockeye` in the package `nlrwr`. The data frame `sockeye` contains the two variables `recruits` and `spawners` (numbers in thousands). Observation no. 12 is left out of the following analyses because a rock slide occurred that year (Carroll and Ruppert, 1988, p. 141). Figure 6.2 shows the data. We see some increase as stock values get larger, but the variation is clearly increasing as the stock is increasing.

```
> plot(recruits ~ spawners, data = sockeye[-12,
+     ], xlab = "Number of spawners (thousands)",
+     ylab = "Number of recruits (thousands)")
```

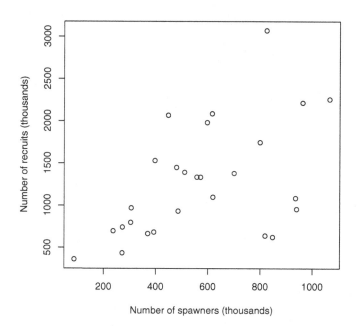

Fig. 6.2. Plot of recruitment as a function of the stock using the dataset sockeye.

Initially we consider a standard nonlinear regression model, assuming variance homogeneity and normality of errors, that is a model of the general form given in Equation (1.3).

```
> sockeye.m1 <- nls(recruits ~ beta1 *
+     spawners * exp(-beta2 * spawners),
+     data = sockeye[-12, ], start = list(beta1 = 2,
+         beta2 = 0.001))
```

The first thing to do is to check the model. Following the approach outlined in Chapter 5, we find that according to the plot of the raw residuals versus the fitted values (not shown), the model seems to capture the systematic deviation in the data quite well, so the chosen mean function appears to be alright. Similarly, the QQ plot (not shown) does not suggest any severe deviation from the normality assumption. On the other hand, the plot of the fitted values versus the absolute residuals in Fig. 6.3 clearly indicates variance heterogeneity: The variation in the absolute residuals is increasing as the fitted values increase.

```
> plot(fitted(sockeye.m1), abs(residuals(sockeye.m1)),
+     xlab = "Fitted values", ylab = "Absolute residuals")
```

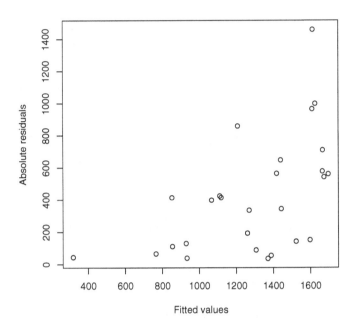

Fig. 6.3. Plot of the fitted values versus the absolute residuals for the model fit sockeye.m1 of the Ricker model to the dataset sockeye (without using a transformation).

So the presence of variance heterogeneity is the only severe deviation from the model assumptions in Section 5.1. We can cope with this model violation by using a variance model (as seen in the previous section) or a transformation. Following Carroll and Ruppert (1988, pp. 139–152), we use a transformation.

In linear regression, it is common to transform the response only (that would be the variable recruits in our example) but otherwise not change the model (Carroll and Ruppert, 1988, p. 117). The same approach can be applied to nonlinear regression models, but it will distort the original relationship between the response and the predictor dictated by the chosen mean function. We insist on preserving this relationship because there is almost always a good reason why a particular mean function is used. Therefore, it is necessary to consider a transform-both-sides approach where both the left- and right-hand sides in Equation (1.1) are transformed

$$h(y) = h\big(f(x, \beta)\big)$$

by using some transformation h (we will get more concrete below). This model ensures that the original relationship between response and predictor is retained, as both the response (left-hand side) and the mean function (right-hand side) are subject to the same transformation. Consequently, the transformed Ricker model can be specified using the following mean function:

$$h\Big(f\big(S, (\alpha, k)\big)\Big) = h\big(\alpha S \exp(kS)\big) + \varepsilon \qquad (6.4)$$

For the right choice of the transformation h, we could hope to achieve that the errors ε are normally distributed with constant variance. How do we find the right transformation?

6.2.2 Finding an appropriate transformation

In practice the transformation h is often estimated from the data unless some apparent choice of transformation is natural for a given dataset (see Exercise 6.4). In order to estimate a transformation, we start out considering a family of transformations that is indexed by a parameter λ, say, such that each value of λ corresponds to another transformation. In this way, estimation of a transformation is simply a matter of estimating a single parameter. The most used family of transformations are the Box-Cox transformations (Box and Cox, 1964), defined as follows:

$$h_\lambda(y) = \begin{cases} \frac{y^\lambda - 1}{\lambda} & \lambda \neq 0 \\ \\ \log(y) & \lambda = 0 \end{cases} \qquad (6.5)$$

For $\lambda = 0$, the logarithm transformation is obtained. For λ different from 0, the Box-Cox transformations are power functions. Well-known transformations included are the reciprocal transformation ($\lambda = -1$), the cubic-root transformation ($\lambda = 1/3$), the square-root transformation ($\lambda = 1/2$), and the quadratic transformation ($\lambda = 2$). The value $\lambda = 1$ is equivalent to not transforming at all, and this fact provides a means for carrying out a hypothesis test to assess whether or not there is a need for a transformation.

One way is to estimate the parameters β in the mean function and λ jointly using a profile likelihood approach (Carroll and Ruppert, 1988, pp. 124–127). This approach is implemented in the `boxcox` method for `nls()` model fits (available in the package `nlrwr`). By default, the `boxcox` method produces a plot of the profile log likelihood function: For a grid of λ values between -2 and 2 (the default interval), the transformed model based on the transformation h_λ is fitted, and the resulting log likelihood values are plotted against the λ

values. Beware: The resulting transformation may not always be successful in establishing normally distributed responses with constant variance.

The optimal transformation within the Box-Cox family for the Ricker model is conveniently done using `boxcox.nls()`, as only the `nls()` model fit needs to be supplied. The resulting plot of the profile log likelihood function for the parameter λ is shown in Fig. 6.4. The estimate of the λ value lies between -1 and 0.

```
> sockeye.m2 <- boxcox.nls(sockeye.m1)
```

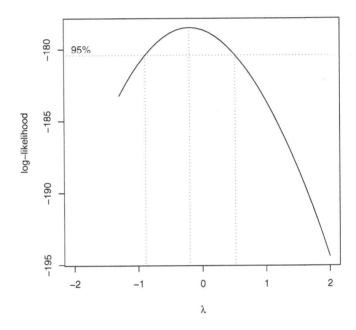

Fig. 6.4. Plot of the profile log likelihood function for the parameter λ for the transform-both-sides Box-Cox transformed Ricker model fitted to the dataset **sockeye**.

Using the function `bcSummary()`, we can extract the estimate of λ together with a 95% confidence interval (the default).

```
> bcSummary(sockeye.m2)

Estimated lambda: -0.2
Confidence interval for lambda: [-0.89, 0.52]
```

So the estimate of λ is -0.2, and the optimal Box-Cox transformation is $h_{-0.2}$ (with reference to Equation (6.5)); that is, a power function with exponent -0.2. The confidence interval does not include $\lambda = 1$, implying that not transforming is not an option. We also see from the confidence interval that $\lambda = 0$ cannot be rejected, meaning that we could also choose to use the logarithm transformation instead of $h_{-0.2}$.

In order to compare the standard errors between the models with and without transformation, the summary output of both sockeye.m1 and sockeye.m2 are needed.

```
> coef(summary(sockeye.m1))

        Estimate     Std. Error   t value
beta1 3.9495589029 1.0154151168 3.889600
beta2 0.0008525523 0.0003570088 2.388043
        Pr(>|t|)
beta1 0.0006575081
beta2 0.0248117796

> coef(summary(sockeye.m2))

        Estimate     Std. Error   t value
beta1 3.7767884397 0.6941023788 5.441256
beta2 0.0009539344 0.0003061565 3.115839
        Pr(>|t|)
beta1 1.195245e-05
beta2 4.563495e-03
```

The parameter estimates are almost the same for both model fits, but the estimated standard errors have changed substantially, becoming smaller as a consequence of applying the transformation.

6.3 Sandwich estimators

Consider a nonlinear regression model specified by Equation (1.3), where the conditional mean structure (Equation (1.2)) imposed by the chosen mean function f is correctly specified but the assumptions regarding normality and/or the variance homogeneity are not satisfied. In this case, the estimated standard errors from the model assuming normality and variance homogeneity will be inconsistent: They will not approach the true standard errors as the sample size increases (Carroll and Ruppert, 1988, p. 128). However, even though the model is misspecified with regard to some of the distributional assumptions, it is still possible to obtain consistent estimates of the standard errors by adjusting the estimated variance-covariance matrix (Carroll and Ruppert, 1988, p. 128). Equation (2.5) is only valid if the model is correctly specified (w.r.t.

both the mean structure and the distributional assumptions). Rewinding the derivation leading to Equation (2.5) the equation

$$\widehat{\text{var}}(\hat{\beta}) = s^2 \hat{B} \hat{M} \hat{B} \tag{6.6}$$

is obtained, where the matrix $\hat{M}$ is a function of the first derivatives of the log likelihood function and $\hat{B}$ is defined as in Equation (2.5). This equation is valid as long as the mean structure is correct and independence can be assumed. Therefore, the resulting estimated variance-covariance matrix is said to be robust against misspecification of the distributional assumptions. If the model is correctly specified, we have the equality $\hat{M} = \hat{B}^{-1}$, and Equation (6.6) reduces to Equation (2.5). The robust variance-covariance matrix is often called a sandwich estimator due to the particular product form on the right-hand side of Equation (6.6), whereas the estimated nonrobust variance-covariance matrix is referred to as naïve. More detailed explanations can be found in White (1981), Carroll and Ruppert (1988, pp. 209–213), White (1996, Chapter 5), and Zeileis (2006). In conclusion, the use of sandwich estimates is attractive, because we avoid having to find a transformation or specify a variance model but can still adjust for deviations from the model assumptions.

For the model fit `sockeye.m1`, the estimated naïve variance-covariance matrix is obtained with the `vcov` method.

```
> vcov(sockeye.m1)
```

```
         beta1        beta2
beta1 1.0310678594 3.436056e-04
beta2 0.0003436056 1.274553e-07
```

The diagonal elements in this matrix are the squared estimated standard errors of the parameter estimates (reported in the corresponding summary output), whereas the off-diagonal elements are estimates of the covariances between parameter estimates. In passing, we note that the `vcov` method can be useful for assessing how strongly correlated the parameter estimates are. High correlation between some of the parameters may indicate that possibly a model with fewer parameters should be considered.

In order to calculate the sandwich estimator, the function `sandwich()` in the package `sandwich` (Zeileis, 2006) can be applied:

```
> sandwich(sockeye.m1)
```

```
         beta1        beta2
beta1 0.6082739547 2.458975e-04
beta2 0.0002458975 1.162302e-07
```

We notice that the elements in the matrix change somewhat. The next step is to look at the summary output to see the actual changes in the estimated standard errors. In order to view the part of the summary output containing parameter estimates and corresponding standard errors, t-tests, and p-values, we could apply the `coef` method to the summary output (as seen in Subsection 6.2.2). Alternatively, we could use the function `coeftest()` in the package `lmtest` (Zeileis and Hothorn, 2002).

The parameter estimates with naive standard errors (using the elements in `vcov(sockeye.m1)`) are shown below.

```
> coeftest(sockeye.m1)

t test of coefficients:

         Estimate Std. Error t value  Pr(>|t|)
beta1 3.94955890 1.01541512  3.8896 0.0006575 ***
beta2 0.00085255 0.00035701  2.3880 0.0248118 *
---
Signif. codes:  0 '***' 0.001 '**' 0.01 '*' 0.05 '.' 0.1 ' ' 1
```

The output is identical to what we get using `coef(summary(sockeye.m1))`. To obtain the estimated standard errors based on the sandwich estimator we can use `coeftest()` again, but this time also specifying the argument `vcov` with the value `sandwich`.

```
> coeftest(sockeye.m1, vcov = sandwich)

t test of coefficients:

         Estimate Std. Error t value  Pr(>|t|)
beta1 3.94955890 0.77991920  5.0641 3.158e-05 ***
beta2 0.00085255 0.00034093  2.5007   0.01931 *
---
Signif. codes:  0 '***' 0.001 '**' 0.01 '*' 0.05 '.' 0.1 ' ' 1
```

Comparing the two outputs, we see that the adjustment leads to a substantially smaller standard error for the parameter β_1, but it does not change the standard error for the parameter β_2 much. The standard error for β_1 based on the sandwich estimator is close to the corresponding standard error obtained from the transformation model `sockeye.m2`. As there may be appreciable differences in the standard errors between the different approaches, we would suggest using the sandwich estimator if there are any doubts about the validity of the distributional assumptions.

6.4 Weighting

Weights can also be used to get the variance structure right, but weights should preferably be used in cases where data have been summarised into averages! If the complete original dataset is available, then there are often better ways to take the variance structure into account (Carroll and Ruppert, 1988, p. 12), as seen in the previous sections.

It happens that the complete dataset is not available to the data analyst because response values have been averaged at some level. Typically, the average response was calculated for each unique predictor value. Ideally, the corresponding empirical standard deviations and the number of replicates for each unique predictor value should also be available because these values can be used to construct weights to be used in the estimation procedure. Denote the weights $w_1, \ldots, w_n$. We consider the following nonlinear regression model:

$$y_i = f(x_i, \beta) + \varepsilon_i / \sqrt{w_i} \tag{6.7}$$

The expectation of y_i is still $f(x_i, \beta)$ (as it was defined in Equation (1.3)), but the variance is now σ^2 / w_i due to the weight introduced in the error term. Through multiplication with $\sqrt{w_i}$, the model in Equation (6.7) can be converted to an equivalent model with error terms (ε_is) that have constant variance σ^2 such that least-squares estimation can be applied. We need not do any multiplication manually. Instead we can use nls() with the weights argument specified to be the variable that corresponds to the w_is (not the $\sqrt{w_i}$s!). Thus estimation in the nonlinear regression model defined in Equation (6.7) amounts to minimising the weighted RSS defined below.

$$\text{weighted RSS}(\beta) = \sum_{i=1}^{n} w_i \big(y_i - f(x_i, \beta)\big)^2$$

Let us return to the average responses. If we assume that there is variance homogeneity (of the original responses, which are averages), then the general model given by Equation (1.3) implies the following variance for the average response ($\overline{y}_i$):

$$\text{var}(\overline{y}_i) = \sigma^2 / m_i$$

So using the number of replicates $m_1, \ldots, m_n$ as weights will result in a model for $\overline{y}_i$ of the form given in Equation (6.7).

If we cannot assume variance homogeneity, we also need to consider the standard deviations (in addition to the number of replicates). In this case, Equation (1.3) implies the following variance:

$$\text{var}(\overline{y}_i) = \sigma_i^2 / m_i$$

We would expect the ratios σ_i^2 / s_i^2 to be roughly 1 because s_i^2 is an estimate of σ_i^2, and multiplication of $\overline{y}_i$ by the weights $\sqrt{m_i} / s_i$ would result in quantities approximately having constant variance 1. Therefore, using the weights $(s_i / \sqrt{m_i})^{-1}$ will result in a model where variance homogeneity is not entirely unreasonable. Be aware that the reasoning above relies heavily on the s_i^2s being good estimates of the σ_i^2s.

If the weights supplied are all the same, then only the estimated residual variance will be influenced (it is merely a scaling), whereas unequal weights will influence the estimated residual variance as well as parameter estimates and estimated standard errors.

6.4.1 Decline in nitrogen content in soil

Laberge et al. (2006) consider two experiments where the decline of nitrogen content from pea residues was followed in soil over 16.5 years. The two experiments correspond to two different ways in which the residues were added to the soil. The resulting datasets are available as exp1 and exp2 in the package nlrwr. Let us consider experiment 1 first. The corresponding dataset is shown below.

```
> exp1

   time Nremaining stdev norep
1  0.08   75.16000  2.61     3
2  0.25   70.07000  2.61     3
3  0.55   60.13000  5.23     3
4  1.00   39.54000  4.58     3
5  2.00   36.00000  1.63     3
6  3.01   29.74000  5.88     3
7  8.64   20.82000  1.26     3
8 16.51   16.20837  2.86     3
```

There are four variables in exp1:

- time is the time elapsed in years (predictor)
- Nremaining is the average percentage of nitrogen available (response)
- stdev is the corresponding standard deviation
- norep is the number of replicates

The data have been summarised for each unique value of the predictor (time). The standard deviations (in the third column) are not varying that much, being of the same order of magnitude, indicating that the assumption of variance homogeneity may be acceptable. A plot of the data is shown in Fig. 6.5.

The model suggested for this type of data is the biexponential model with mean function

$$f(\text{time}, (a_1, a_2, b_1, b_2)) = a_1 \exp(-\exp(a_2)\text{time}) + b_1 \exp(-\exp(b_2)\text{time})$$

The reason for choosing this model is that it is anticipated that there are several mechanisms involved, causing exponential decays at different rates (Laberge et al., 2006). A self-starter function is available for the biexponential model: SSbiexp() (see Table B.1 in Appendix B). First, we fit the model where each average response is treated as a single response value, ignoring the number of replicates and standard deviations. Next, we fit the same model, but this time using the appropriate weights (norep/(stdev*stdev)).

```
> plot(Nremaining ~ time, data = exp1,
+     xlab = "Time (years)", ylab = "Nitrogen content (%)")
```

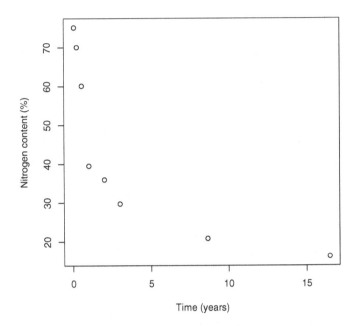

Fig. 6.5. Decline in nitrogen content over time for experiment 1.

```
> exp1.m1 <- nls(Nremaining ~ SSbiexp(time,
+     a1, a2, b1, b2), data = exp1)
> exp1.m2 <- nls(Nremaining ~ SSbiexp(time,
+     a1, a2, b1, b2), data = exp1,
+     weights = norep/(stdev * stdev))
```

The actual values of the weights can be retrieved using the `weights` method.

```
> weights(exp1.m2)
```

```
[1] 0.4403928 0.4403928 0.1096776
[4] 0.1430179 1.1291355 0.0867694
[7] 1.8896447 0.3667661
```

A comparison of the two model fits by means of their summary output looks as follows (notice the use of the `coef` method applied to the summary output in order to get a more concise output):

```
> coef(summary(exp1.m1))
```

```
   Estimate Std. Error    t value     Pr(>|t|)
a1 49.6945735  6.1714388  8.0523481 0.001291449
a2  0.2182533  0.3162611  0.6901049 0.528080831
b1 32.2059455  6.1631160  5.2255946 0.006402928
b2 -3.1242900  0.4881789 -6.3998879 0.003061147

> coef(summary(exp1.m2))

    Estimate Std. Error     t value    Pr(>|t|)
a1 48.95580529  5.8454395  8.37504275 0.001111764
a2 -0.02288415  0.2953566 -0.07747973 0.941962763
b1 30.67388498  6.4550371  4.75193009 0.008958175
b2 -3.15057479  0.5205589 -6.05229290 0.003760909
```

We see that the parameter estimates change only slightly, except for a2, which differs considerably between the two model fits. There also are only slight changes in the estimated standard errors. This is not surprising, as the weights supplied are of roughly the same magnitude.

The dataset exp2 is similar to exp1 with respect to the variables included. However, the standard deviations vary substantially (several orders of magnitude).

```
> exp2

   time Nremaining stdev norep
1  0.08   92.48000 10.46     3
2  0.25   75.49000  5.23     3
3  0.55   74.51000  7.19     3
4  1.00   60.13000 10.46     3
5  2.00   50.00000  2.61     3
6  3.01   45.42000  0.01     3
7  7.64   26.94000  1.64     3
8 15.51   17.14786  2.50     3
```

Again we fit biexponential models with and without weights using nls() and the self-starter SSbiexp().

```
> exp2.m1 <- nls(Nremaining ~ SSbiexp(time,
+       a1, a2, b1, b2), data = exp2)
> exp2.m2 <- nls(Nremaining ~ SSbiexp(time,
+       a1, a2, b1, b2), data = exp2,
+       weights = norep/(stdev^2))
```

The estimated regression curves are shown in Fig. 6.6. The curves appear to be quite similar.

```
> plot(Nremaining ~ time, data = exp2,
+       xlab = "Time (years)", ylab = "Nitrogen content (%)")
```

```
> timeVal <- with(exp2, seq(min(time),
+     max(time), length.out = 100))
> lines(timeVal, predict(exp2.m1,
+     newdata = data.frame(time = timeVal)),
+     lty = 2)
> lines(timeVal, predict(exp2.m2,
+     newdata = data.frame(time = timeVal)),
+     lty = 3)
```

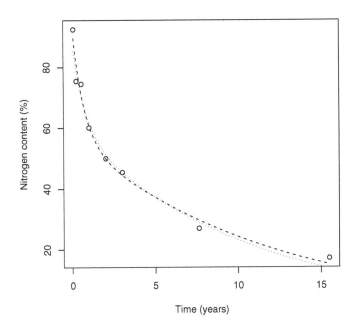

Fig. 6.6. Decline in nitrogen content over time for experiment 2 (the dataset `exp2`) together with estimated regression curves based on model fits without and with weights, respectively.

Looking at the summary outputs, we find that the parameter estimates change moderately, whereas three out of four estimated standard errors change quite dramatically (by a factor of 2) as a consequence of using the weights.

```
> coef(summary(exp2.m1))

      Estimate Std. Error    t value    Pr(>|t|)
a1 37.1828528  7.3946626  5.0283366 0.007342087
```

```
a2   0.3984263   0.4676840     0.8519135 0.442262764
b1  56.9940957   7.2995778     7.8078619 0.001451984
b2  -2.4593036   0.2429193   -10.1239547 0.000535818

> coef(summary(exp2.m2))

    Estimate Std. Error      t value       Pr(>|t|)
a1 28.9158392  8.3745109    3.4528392 2.598700e-02
a2  0.3128281  0.8122243    0.3851499 7.197304e-01
b1 59.7777230  3.7595533   15.9002197 9.144765e-05
b2 -2.3567707  0.1311759  -17.9664898 5.641332e-05
```

Moreover, the estimated residual error in the summary output of the model fit exp2.m2 (not shown) is not as far from 1, as we would expect after applying the weights.

Exercises

6.1. Consider the dataset RGRcurve. Fit the two-parameter exponential model, but in such a way that the variance is assumed to be an exponential function of the mean.

6.2. Verify for the model fit sockeye.m1 that the mean structure is appropriate and that the normality assumption is acceptable.

6.3. Consider the dataset sockeye. Fit the Ricker model, but this time with a variance model included. Compare the results to the fits sockeye.m1 and sockeye.m2 and to the results based on the sandwich estimator.

6.4. Fit the exponential model (Equation (3.2)) to the dataset O.mykiss. Check the model assumptions. Are there any problems? For this kind of data, it is common to apply a transform-both-sides approach using the logarithm transformation (OECD (Organisation for Economic Cooperation and Development), 2006b), so in this case there is no need to look for the best transformation. Fit the logarithm-transformed model, and check the model assumptions. Is there any improvement over the initial fit?

7

Uncertainty, Hypothesis Testing, and Model Selection

Nonlinear regression methods often rely on the assumption that the nonlinear mean function can be approximated by a linear function locally. This linear approximation may or may not be used in the estimation algorithm (e.g., the Gauss-Newton algorithm), but more importantly it is often used to obtain standard errors, confidence intervals, and t-tests, all of which will depend on how good the approximation is.

The quality of the linear approximation can be summarised by means of two features of the model referred to as intrinsic curvature and parameter effects curvature. We will not provide rigorous definitions here. More details can be found in Bates and Watts (1988, Chapter 7). The two curvature measures reflect different aspects of the linear approximation: (1) The planar assumption ensures that it is possible to approximate the nonlinear mean function at a given point using a tangent plane. (2) The uniform coordinate assumption means that a linear coordinate system is imposed on the approximating tangent plane. Intrinsic curvature is related to the planar assumption, and it depends on the dataset considered and the mean function but not on the parameterisation used in the mean function. Parameter effects curvature is related to the uniform coordinate assumption, and it depends on all aspects of the model, including the parameterisation. Large values of these two curvature measures indicate a poor linear approximation. The function rms.curv() in the package MASS can be used to calculate the two measures for a given nls() model fit (Venables and Ripley, 2002b).

In many cases the intrinsic curvature will be negligible compared with the parameter effects curvature (Bates and Watts, 1988, p. 256), and in such cases the profile likelihood approach in Section 7.1 is likely to be useful. The bootstrap approach in Section 7.2 is another alternative. The Wald procedures in Sections 7.3 and 7.4 are influenced by both intrinsic curvature and parameter effects curvature, and therefore they should be used with some reservation, especially for small datasets. Sections 7.5 and 7.6 consider comparisons between nested and non-nested models, respectively.

7.1 Profile likelihood

For a parameter of interest, say β_j, the profile t function is defined as

$$\tau(\beta_j) = \text{sign}(\beta_j - \hat{\beta}_j) \frac{\sqrt{\text{RSS}(\beta_j) - \text{RSS}(\hat{\beta})}}{s} \tag{7.1}$$

where the profile RSS function β_j (that is, $\text{RSS}(\beta_j)$ in Equation (7.1)) is defined in Subsection 4.3.2 and s denotes the residual standard error defined in Section 2.1. The profile t function can be used to examine the extent of curvature in the direction of the parameter β_j. More details on the profiling approach can be found in Bates and Watts (1988, Section 6.1) and Venables and Ripley (2002a, Section 8.4).

The `profile` method, applicable to any model fit obtained using `nls()`, will calculate the profile t function for each parameter in the model unless otherwise specified (see below). In fact, the only argument needed in `profile` is the model fit. Before we do the profiling, we use the `update` method to fit `L.minor.m1`, but this time switching off the trace (it was switched on in Subsection 2.2.2) to avoid the subsequent profiling, which involves refitting the model several times over a grid of β_j values, to fill the **R** console with trace output.

```
> L.minor.m1 <- update(L.minor.m1,
+     trace = FALSE)
> L.minor.m1pro <- profile(L.minor.m1)
```

Profiling is done for all parameters in the model (use the argument `which` to limit the profiling to fewer parameters). To show the profile t functions for the parameters in the model, the corresponding `plot` method can be applied to profiling result `L.minor.m1pro`. The resulting plot is shown in Fig. 7.1. By default, the absolute value of $\tau(\beta_j)$ is plotted as a function of the parameter being profiled.

```
> plot(L.minor.m1pro)
```

To obtain plots using the original $\tau(\beta_j)$ values instead of absolute values, the argument `absVal` can be used. It takes a logical value (`FALSE` or `TRUE`) to specify the absence or presence of absolute values. The resulting plot is shown in Fig. 7.2.

```
> plot(L.minor.m1pro, absVal = FALSE)
```

The plots in both Fig. 7.1 and Fig. 7.2 show that there is some curvature for the parameter K, indicating that the linear approximation is not perfect in that parameter component. In contrast, the linear approximation seems quite acceptable for the parameter V_m, as there is only very slight curvature for this parameter component.

Profile confidence intervals, which are obtained by referring $\tau(\beta_j)$ in Equation (tau) to the appropriate percentiles in a t-distribution with $n - p$ degrees of freedom, are extracted using the confint method. The 95% confidence intervals of the two parameters in L.minor.m1 are shown below.

```
> confint(L.minor.m1)

       2.5%      97.5%
K    11.45520   24.86789
Vm  110.64411  143.75862
```

The argument level can be used to specify the confidence level(s) required. We could already have read off the intervals from Fig. 7.1 or Fig. 7.2 using the solid vertical lines dropped from the profile function onto the x axis. By

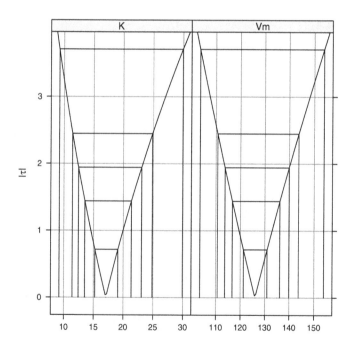

Fig. 7.1. Plots of the profile t functions for the two parameters K and V_m in the Michaelis-Menten model fitted to the dataset L.minor.

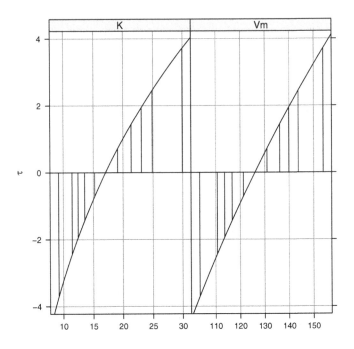

Fig. 7.2. Plots of the profile t functions (using the untransformed τ values) for the two parameters in the Michaelis-Menten model fitted to the dataset L.minor.

default, 50%, 80%, 90%, 95%, and 99% confidence intervals are shown on the plots of the profile functions, but this can be controlled by means of the argument conf for specifying the desired confidence levels.

7.2 Bootstrap

An alternative to profile confidence intervals is to apply the bootstrap to repeatedly generate datasets based on the fitted nonlinear regression model. Confidence intervals based on the bootstrap approach do not rely on the linear approximation.

We will use the function nlsBoot() in the package nlstools and the associated plot and summary methods. This means that we use a nonparametric bootstrap approach where the mean centered residuals are bootstrapped (Venables and Ripley, 2002a, Chapter 8). By default, nlsBoot() generates 999 datasets, and for each dataset the original nonlinear regression model is fitted and the resulting parameter estimates stored. We store the bootstrap results generated by nlsBoot() when applied to the model fit L.minor.m1 in the object L.minor.m1boot.

```
> L.minor.m1boot <- nlsBoot(L.minor.m1)
```

The bootstrapped values are useful for assessing the marginal distributions of the parameter estimates, so we start out by comparing them with a normal distribution, which they should ideally follow if the linear approximation holds. To this end, we can use normal QQ plots, which we already used in Subsection 5.4.1. The resulting plots are shown in Fig. 7.3. The points in the two normal QQ plots in Fig. 7.3 do not follow a straight line exactly, showing some curvature, especially in the tails some departure from the normal distribution is apparent.

To obtain bootstrap confidence intervals, the **summary** method is used. The confidence intervals obtained are so-called percentile confidence intervals that are based on percentiles in the empirical distribution of the bootstrap parameter estimates. If 999 bootstrap simulations are used, then the empirical distribution is based on 1000 values: the original estimate and the 999 bootstrap estimates. Thus, to construct a 95% percentile confidence interval, we take the 25th value and the 975th value among the 1000 ordered estimates (ordered from smallest to largest) as left and right endpoints, respectively. The percentile confidence interval has the advantage of lying entirely within the range of plausible parameter values, which in the case of the Michaelis-Menten model means the range from 0 upwards. This is in contrast to Wald confidence intervals (Section 7.3), which for small samples occasionally may give unrealistic lower and upper limits. The 95% bootstrap confidence intervals for the parameters K and V_m are shown below.

```
> summary(L.minor.m1boot)

------
Bootstrap estimates
       K        Vm
17.27010 125.89618


------
Bootstrap confidence intervals
      2.5%     97.5%

> qqnorm(L.minor.m1boot$coefboot[,
+     1], main = "K")
> qqnorm(L.minor.m1boot$coefboot[,
+     2], main = "Vm")
```

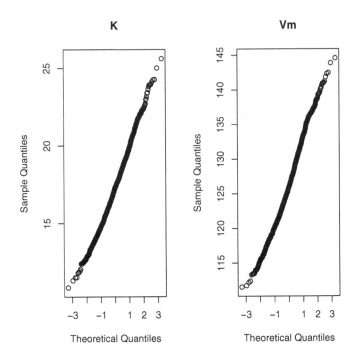

Fig. 7.3. Normal QQ plots of the 999 bootstrap parameter estimates for each of the two parameters K and V_m in the Michaelis-Menten model fitted to the dataset *L.minor*.

```
K    12.88137   22.32728
Vm 115.58938  138.58658
```

The 95% percentile confidence intervals are slightly narrower than the profile confidence intervals obtained in Section 7.1. It is also worth noting that the intervals are slightly asymmetric, as was in fact also the case for the profile confidence intervals. In conclusion, the bootstrap and profile likelihood confidence intervals of the analysis of L.minor agree quite well. Apart from the bootstrap confidence intervals, the summary of the bootstrap results also shows the median values of bootstrap estimates for each parameter, which can be used to assess if there is any bias present in the parameter estimates. This seems not to be the case here (comparing the values above to the original parameter estimates 17.08 and 126.0).

Another example using the bootstrap approach is found in Venables and Ripley (2002a, Section 8.4).

The bootstrap approach is somewhat computer-intensive, as the nonlinear regression model considered has to be refitted numerous times, but for many applications it will still be a feasible approach. Moreover, the linear approximation will improve as the sample size increases, and therefore the bootstrap approach may be most useful for small datasets.

7.3 Wald confidence intervals

In this section, we consider confidence intervals that are based on asymptotic or large sample results, which may not necessarily work well for small sample sizes where the linear approximation may be poor. Denote the estimated asymptotic standard error of the parameter estimate $\hat{\beta}_j$ by $se(\hat{\beta}_j)$. The $1 - \alpha$ Wald confidence interval of the parameter β_j is then defined as

$$\hat{\beta}_j \pm t_{1-\alpha/2,n-p} se(\hat{\beta}_j)$$

where $t_{1-\alpha/2,n-p}$ denotes the $1 - \alpha/2$ percentile in a t-distribution with $n - p$ degrees of freedom. Several approximations are at work in this definition. The linear approximation is used to obtain $se(\hat{\beta}_j)$, and the use of a t-distribution is also only an approximation. However, these confidence intervals may still be useful in applications. We have seen examples where they work well for models with 3–5 parameters and sample sizes as small as 20–30, but, in general, you should exert caution in relying on these confidence intervals.

The Wald confidence intervals for the two parameters K and V_m based on the model fit L.minor.m1 can be retrieved from the model fit using the confint2 method from the package nlrwr in the following way:

```
> confint2(L.minor.m1)

        2.5 %     97.5 %
K     9.853828   24.30416
Vm  108.480813  143.58470
```

In this case, the resulting confidence intervals do not differ much from the confidence intervals based on the profiling and bootstrap approaches. To get confidence intervals for other confidence levels, the argument level needs to be specified. For example, the following line produces the 99% confidence intervals of the parameters.

```
> confint2(L.minor.m1, level = 0.99)

        0.5 %     99.5 %
K     6.131815   28.02617
Vm  99.439005  152.62651
```

7.4 Estimating derived parameters

If we can assume that the joint distribution of the parameter estimates approximately follows a normal distribution, which is again a matter of the validity of the linear approximation, then it follows that any smooth (that is, differentiable) transformation of the parameter estimates will again be approximately normally distributed.

In more detail, assume that the parameter estimates $\hat{\beta}$ are approximately normally distributed with a variance-covariance matrix estimated by $V(\hat{\beta})$, which we can get from an nls() model fit using the vcov method. Then the derived parameter $g(\hat{\beta})$, which is a function g of the original parameter estimates $\hat{\beta}$, is again approximately normally distributed with an estimated variance-covariance matrix $Dg(\hat{\beta})^t V(\hat{\beta}) Dg(\hat{\beta})$, where $Dg(\hat{\beta})$ denotes the gradient of g; that is, the vector of first derivatives of g with respect to the parameters evaluated at the parameter estimates $\hat{\beta}$ (van der Vaart, 1998, Chapter 3). Bailer and Piegorsch (2000, p. 88) and Weisberg (2005, pp. 120–122) provide some good examples that explain this approach in more detail. This result is extremely powerful, as it makes it possible to establish approximate normality for various derived parameters, that are functions of the original parameters in the model. Applying this result is usually referred to as using the delta method. Of course, if the original parameter estimates are not approximately normally distributed, then the delta method will not work well. In such cases, it may be better to use a bootstrap approach, generating a bootstrap estimate of the derived parameter of interest for each bootstrap estimate of the original parameters and then proceeding along the lines of Section 7.2. Next, we will show how to use the delta method in **R**.

As a measure of the rate of change of the underlying enzymatic process, it can be useful to consider the slope of the Michaelis-Menten curve at the concentration K: The larger the slope, the faster the enzymatic reaction goes. The slope of the curve at the concentration K is a function of the two parameters K and V_m:

$$\frac{V_m}{4K} \tag{7.2}$$

The estimate of the slope is calculated by plugging in the parameter estimates of K and V_m in Equation (7.2), but how do we obtain the corresponding estimated standard error? We use the delta method!

The function to use in **R** is delta.method() in the package alr3. We need to supply two arguments to this function: first, the model fit from which to retrieve the parameter estimates and the estimated variance-covariance matrix, and second, the expression of the derived parameter to be calculated (as a string, in quotation marks). For the model fit L.minor.m1, the specification looks like this:

```
> delta.method(L.minor.m1, "Vm/(4*K)")
```

Functions of parameters: expression(Vm/(4 * K))
Estimate = 1.844850 with se = 0.2363011

Thus we find that the rate of change is estimated to be 1.84, and the corresponding estimated standard error is 0.24.

7.5 Nested models

Let us assume that we have fitted a nonlinear regression model that provides an adequate description of a given dataset. Then, the next step would often be to try to simplify the model in order to obtain the most parsimonious description of the data. Simplification could mean that some of the parameters in the model are replaced by fixed values such that eventually fewer parameters are used to describe the data. In the terminology of Equation (1.3), we consider the null hypothesis

$$H_0 : \beta_j = \beta_{0j} \tag{7.3}$$

for some parameter of interest β_j and for some given value β_{0j}.

In the following two subsections, we will discuss two ways of testing the null hypothesis. We will use the data frame secalonic in the package drc to illustrate the different approaches. The data in secalonic stem from a large experiment exploring the toxicity of secalonic acid to roots of various grasses (Gong et al., 2004). The data are shown below.

```
> secalonic

    dose rootl
1 0.000   5.5
2 0.010   5.7
3 0.019   5.4
4 0.038   4.6
5 0.075   3.3
6 0.150   0.7
7 0.300   0.4
```

The dataset contains a response variable (rootl), which is the root length (in cm), and a predictor variable (dose), which is the dose of secalonic acid applied (in mM). The response values are means of an unknown number of replicates. Figure 7.4 shows the data.

The dose-response relationship is clearly sigmoidal, and therefore the four-parameter logistic model is a natural choice (Streibig et al., 1993). The logistic model is conveniently fitted using the self-starter SSfpl() (see Table B.1 in Appendix B).

```
> secalonic.m1 <- nls(rootl ~ SSfpl(dose,
+      a, b, c, d), data = secalonic)
```

```
> plot(rootl ~ dose, data = secalonic,
+     xlab = "Dose (mM)", ylab = "Root length (cm)")
```

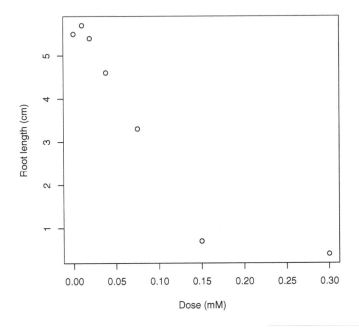

Fig. 7.4. Plot of the root length as a function of the dose of secalonic acid based on the dataset `secalonic`.

In the next two subsections, we will show how to carry out hypothesis testing using the model fit `secalonic.m1` as the starting point.

7.5.1 Using *t*-tests

To test the null hypothesis in Equation (7.3) with $\beta_{0j} = 0$ (that is, testing whether or not the parameter is equal to 0), we can use the *t*-test statistic

$$t = \frac{\hat{\beta}_j - \beta_{0j}}{se(\hat{\beta}_j)} = \frac{\hat{\beta}_j}{se(\hat{\beta}_j)} \tag{7.4}$$

which is the difference between the parameter estimate $\hat{\beta}_j$ and the given value β_{0j} divided by the corresponding estimated standard error $se(\hat{\beta}_j)$. The test statistic *t* approximately follows a *t*-distribution with $n - p$ degrees of freedom. Using the `summary` method, we can instantaneously get *t*-tests based on Equation (7.4) with the corresponding *p*-values for all parameters in the model. Typically only one or a few – if any – of these hypotheses are relevant to consider. Let us have a look at the summary output for the model fit secalonic.m1.

```
> summary(secalonic.m1)

Formula: root1 ~ SSfpl(dose, a, b, c, d)

Parameters:
  Estimate Std. Error t value Pr(>|t|)
a 6.053612   0.395467  15.308 0.000606 ***
b 0.353944   0.194089   1.824 0.165722
c 0.075188   0.005911  12.721 0.001048 **
d 0.029350   0.006621   4.433 0.021333 *
---
Signif. codes:  0 '***' 0.001 '**' 0.01 '*' 0.05 '.' 0.1 ' ' 1

Residual standard error: 0.2028 on 3 degrees of freedom

Number of iterations to convergence: 0
Achieved convergence tolerance: 8.101e-06
```

The parameters a and b are the upper and lower limits on the observed root length. The logistic model will predict root lengths close to a for doses almost 0, and the predicted root lengths will approach b as the dose becomes very large. It would be natural to expect that the lower limit will be close to 0, as large doses may prohibit any growth, and therefore it is relevant to consider the hypothesis $H_0 : b = 0$. The value of the corresponding t-test statistic is 1.82. The corresponding p-value based on the t-distribution with 3 degrees of freedom is 0.166. This means that we cannot reject the hypothesis $H_0 : b = 0$, tentatively suggesting that the lower limit could be 0. The result is not surprising in light of Fig. 7.4. Consequently, we can simplify the original four-parameter logistic model by fixing the lower limit at 0 to obtain a three-parameter model describing the data. This three-parameter model is also available in a self-starter version for nls(), namely SSlogis() (we will use it in the next subsection).

A related approach for testing the hypothesis $H_0 : \beta_j = \beta_{j0}$ would be to use confidence intervals: If β_{j0} is not contained in the 95% confidence interval of β_j, then the hypothesis in Equation (7.3) is rejected at a significance level of 5%. So this approach can be applied using either profile, bootstrap, or Wald confidence intervals.

7.5.2 Using F-tests

The t-tests rely on the estimated standard errors and thus rely to a large extent on the linear approximation of the mean function. By using the F-test, we can curb the influence on the linear approximation. In order to apply the F-test, two models need to be fitted: Model A and Model B. Model B should be a submodel of Model A; that is, obtained from Model A by imposing some constraint on the parameters. The choice of submodel will be determined by the null hypothesis that is of interest. The F-test statistic is defined as

$$F = \frac{(\mathrm{RSS_B}(\hat{\beta}_B) - \mathrm{RSS_A}(\hat{\beta}_A))/(df_B - df_A)}{\mathrm{SS_A}/df_A}$$

where subscripts A and B refer to Model A and Model B, respectively. This test statistic is related to the statistic introduced in Subsection 5.2.3. The test is sometimes referred to as the extra-sum-of-squares F-test (Motulsky and Christopoulos, 2004, Chapter 22). The main ingredient in the statistic is the difference between the RSS quantities for the two models considered. A large difference means that the two models are quite different, whereas a small difference indicates that they provide similar fits to the data. Large and small can be quantified by means of a p-value obtained from an F-distribution with degrees of freedom $(df_B - df_A, df_A)$.

Getting back to the dataset `secalonic`, the first step is to fit the submodel that we want to compare to the initial model. Thus we fit the three-parameter logistic model where the lower limit is fixed at 0. The reason for considering this submodel is of that we want to test the hypothesis that the lower limit could be 0 (just as it was in the previous subsection). As already mentioned, the relevant self-starter function is `SSlogis()`.

```
> secalonic.m2 <- nls(root1 ~ SSlogis(dose,
+     a, c, d), data = secalonic)
```

To assess whether or not the reduction from the model fit `secalonic.m1` to the model fit `secalonic.m2` is warranted by the data, the `anova` method is invoked to calculate the F-test defined above.

```
> anova(secalonic.m2, secalonic.m1)
```

```
Analysis of Variance Table

Model 1: root1 ~ SSlogis(dose, a, c, d)
Model 2: root1 ~ SSfpl(dose, a, b, c, d)
  Res.Df Res.Sum Sq Df  Sum Sq F value
1      4    0.25924
2      3    0.12341  1 0.13582  3.3016
  Pr(>F)
1
2 0.1668
```

The order of the arguments `secalonic.m2` and `secalonic.m1` does not have any effect on the resulting p-value, but we still always specify the fitted submodel as the first argument in `anova`. The F-test yields the same conclusion as was already established using the t-test, in fact giving almost the same p-value as the t-test in the previous subsection (see Exercise 7.4 for a situation where results differ).

7.6 Non-nested models

Consider a collection of candidate models that has been chosen a priori for a particular dataset. These models need not be submodels of each other, and therefore it may not be possible to use the F-test procedure introduced in the previous section to compare these models. How then do we decide which model is the most appropriate?

Ideally, the experimenter collecting or generating the data should decide which model to use based on subject matter. If no such suggestions are available, then it may be useful to use some kind of statistic to compare the available models. The basic idea is to calculate the value of the statistic for each candidate model and then compare these values to determine which model provides the best fit. The decision rule is simple: One model is better than another model if it has the smallest value of the statistic. Based on all pairwise comparisons using this rule, a ranking of the candidate models can be established.

The residual standard error and Akaike's information criterion (AIC) (Burnham and Anderson, 2002, pp. 94–96) are two statistics, that are often used for model comparison and selection. The residual standard error is a measure of the distance between the data and fitted regression curve based on the model fit, whereas we can think of the AIC as being an estimate of the distance from the model fit to the true but unknown model that generated the data. The AIC is defined as -2 times the maximum value of the log likelihood plus 2 times the number of parameters in the model. Using Equation (2.4) in Subsection 2.2.2, the AIC can be written as

$$\begin{aligned} \text{AIC} = &-2\log\left(L(\hat{\beta}, \hat{\sigma}^2)\right) + 2(p+1) \\ = & \ n\log(2\pi) + n\log(\text{RSS}(\hat{\beta})/n) + n + 2(p+1) \end{aligned} \qquad (7.5)$$

For nonlinear regression models as defined by Equation (1.3), the AIC is a function of the residual sum of squares, the number of observations and number of parameters (Burnham and Anderson, 2002, p. 94), so the same ingredients are used in both the residual standard error and the AIC, but, as we shall see shortly, they will not in general produce the same ranking of the models. By definition, the AIC includes a penalty for the number of parameters used (the term $2(p+1)$ in Equation (7.5)). Therefore, using the AIC will take the model complexity into account, and this feature may curb overfitting.

We consider the dataset M.merluccius, which contains stock and recruitment data for hake in the period 1982–1996 (see also Section 1.1). Cadima (2003, pp. 47–49) considers four stock-recruitment models for these data:

- Beverton-Holt:
  $$f\big(S, (\alpha, k)\big) = \frac{\alpha S}{1 + S/k} \text{ (introduced in Section 1.1)}$$
- Deriso:
  $$f\big(S, (\alpha, c, k)\big) = \alpha S(1 - \tfrac{cS}{k})^{1/c}$$
- Ricker:
  $$f\big(S, (\alpha, k)\big) = \alpha S \exp(-kS) \text{ (introduced in Subsection 6.2.1)}$$
- Shepherd:
  $$f\big(S, (\alpha, c, k)\big) = \frac{\alpha S}{1 + \left(\frac{S}{k}\right)^c}$$

The Beverton-Holt and Ricker models use two parameters, whereas the Deriso and Shepherd models involve three parameters. For all four models, the parameter α is the slope of the regression curve at $S = 0$. We can fit the models using nls().

```
> M.merluccius.bh <- nls(num.fish ~
+     spawn.biomass * alpha/(1 +
+         spawn.biomass/k), data = M.merluccius,
+     start = list(alpha = 5,
+         k = 50))
> M.merluccius.de <- nls(num.fish ~
+     spawn.biomass * alpha *
+         (1 - c * spawn.biomass/k)^(1/c),
+     data = M.merluccius, start = list(alpha = 4.4,
+         k = 106, c = 0.86))
> M.merluccius.ri <- nls(num.fish ~
+     spawn.biomass * alpha *
+         exp(-spawn.biomass/k),
+     data = M.merluccius, start = list(alpha = 5,
+         k = 50))
> M.merluccius.sh <- nls(num.fish ~
+     spawn.biomass * alpha/(1 +
+         (spawn.biomass/k)^c),
+     data = M.merluccius, start = list(alpha = 3.87,
+         k = 61.72, c = 2.25),
+     control = nls.control(maxiter = 100))
```

In order to obtain convergence in the Shepherd model (M.merluccius.sh), it is necessary to increase the default number of iterations from 50 and up to 100 using the function nls.control() with the argument maxiter.

To extract the estimated residual standard errors from the model fits, we could use the summary output for each model fit, but as we are only interested in a single piece of information in the output, we extract that component directly using $ (use str(summary(M.merluccius.bh)) to get a list of all components in the summary object summary(M.merluccius.bh) and identify the component sigma).

```
> summary(M.merluccius.bh)$sigma

[1] 14.69956

> summary(M.merluccius.de)$sigma

[1] 14.78346

> summary(M.merluccius.ri)$sigma

[1] 14.30425

> summary(M.merluccius.sh)$sigma

[1] 14.56758
```

A comparison of the numbers shows that the Ricker model has the smallest estimated residual standard error, and therefore that would be the model to choose.

The function AIC() can be used to retrieve the AIC value from a model fit. The AIC values for the four stock-recruitment models are obtained as follows, simply supplying the model fit as the only argument to AIC().

```
> AIC(M.merluccius.bh)

[1] 127.0562

> AIC(M.merluccius.de)

[1] 128.0263

> AIC(M.merluccius.ri)

[1] 126.2383

> AIC(M.merluccius.sh)

[1] 127.5850
```

The best model is again found to be the Ricker model, but the mutual ranking of the models has changed as compared with the ranking based on the residual standard errors: The two three-parameter models, the Deriso and Shepherd models, end up having the largest AIC values, being penalised for using one parameter more than the two other models. However, the differences between the AIC values for the four model fits are small when judged by the rule of thumb given in Burnham and Anderson (2002, pp. 70–72), which requires a difference in AIC of more than 10 in order to definitely prefer one model over another model. Therefore we would expect the models to provide very similar descriptions of the dataset M.merluccius.

Exercises

7.1. In Section 4.4, we consider the model fit

```
> RScompetition.m1 <- nls(biomass ~
+     a/(1 + b * (x + c * z)), data = RScompetition,
+     start = list(a = 20, b = 1,
+         c = 1))
```

The interesting parameter is c, and it can be used to quantify the degree of competition between the two biotypes. Obtain a 95% confidence interval for this parameter in order to show the range of plausible values of c.

7.2. Are any of the t-tests reported in the summary output of `L.minor.m1` of interest?

7.3. Compare the Clapeyron and Antoine models for the dataset `vapCO` (Subsection 5.2.1) by means of an F-test.

7.4. The Brain-Cousens model is given by the mean function

$$f\big(x, (b, d, e, f)\big) = \frac{d + fx}{1 + \left(\frac{x}{e}\right)^b} \qquad (7.6)$$

Fit the model to the dataset `lettuce`. The null hypothesis $H_0 : f = 0$ can be interpreted as the absence of a hormetical effect at low concentrations. Is there evidence in the data in favour of rejction of this hypothesis? Test the hypothesis using both a t-test and an F-test. What is the conclusion?

7.5. The data frame `ScotsPine` contains leaf area indices for various ages (in years) collected for a number of Scots pine trees (*Pinus sylvestris L.*). The leaf ratio index is the ratio between the single-sided leaf surface area and the ground surface area. Bailer and Piegorsch (2000, Chapter 2) suggest using the monoexponential model with mean function

$$f\big(\text{age}, (a, b, c)\big) = a + b \cdot \exp(-\text{age}/c) \qquad (7.7)$$

to describe the relationship between age and leaf ratio index. Fit the model and report the 95% confidence intervals for the parameters. Is there anything suspicious?

7.6. Consider the Michaelis-Menten model fit `L.minor.m4` from Section 2.3:

```
> L.minor.m4 <- glm(rate ~ I(1/conc),
+     data = L.minor, family = gaussian(link = "inverse"))
```

The intercept in the model fit corresponds to $\tilde{\beta}_0 = 1/V_m$, and the slope parameter corresponds to $\tilde{\beta}_1 = K/V_m$, which means that we have the following expressions for the original parameters: $V_m = 1/\tilde{\beta}_0$ and $K = \tilde{\beta}_1/\tilde{\beta}_0$. Use the delta method to obtain parameter estimates of the original parameters in the Michaelis-Menten model and the corresponding standard errors.

8

Grouped Data

Often the relationship between response and predictor has been recorded for
several levels of a grouping variable. Examples are:

- enzymatic reaction rates for a range of substrate concentrations recorded
  for each of two treatments
- dry matter weight of plants measured for a number of herbicide doses
  recorded for each of two herbicide treatments

We refer to this type of data as grouped data. One reason for considering
grouped data is that data pertaining to one experiment should be analysed in
one model, as this allows comparisons among groups at various levels.

We start out by considering models assuming variance homogeneity but
now also across groups, which means that the same constant variance applies
to all observations regardless of their group membership. In Section 8.1, we will
show how to fit nonlinear regression models for grouped data, and the topic
in Section 8.2 is model reduction of nonlinear regression models for grouped
data. Sections 8.3 and 8.4 deal with the case of a common control group
for all remaining groups and prediction for grouped-data model, respectively.
Variance homogeneity is not always a reasonable assumption, as there may
be more than one source of variation in play in grouped data structures. We
consider this situation in Section 8.5.

8.1 Fitting grouped data models

In comparison with the situation with only one group, which we dealt with
in the previous chapters, estimation of nonlinear regression models for several treatments requires that the treatment factor is explicitly introduced. In
the following subsections, we will consider a range of ways to fit nonlinear
regression models to grouped data.

The example used throughout this section will be the dataset Puromycin,
which consists of measurements of enzymatic reaction rates for a range of

substrate concentrations. The experiment was carried out with two different treatments: treating the enzyme with the antibiotic puromycin or leaving the enzyme untreated. The response, predictor, and grouping factor are named rate, conc, and state, respectively.

We use the function xyplot() (in the package lattice) to show the data. The resulting scatter plot in Fig. 8.1 shows the data separated by treatment group. There appears to be a marked difference in the upper limit between the two treatments, whereas the concentration producing a reaction rate halfway between 0 and the upper limit could be the same for both treatments.

```
> xyplot(rate ~ conc | state, data = Puromycin,
+     xlab = "Substrate concentration (ppm)",
+     ylab = "Reaction rates\n(counts/min/min)")
```

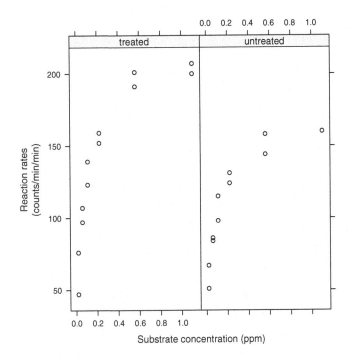

Fig. 8.1. Conditional scatter plot of reaction rate versus substrate concentration for the two groups in the dataset Puromycin.

Following Bates and Watts (1988, pp. 33–34), we consider the Michaelis-Menten model for describing the rate (rate).

$$f\bigl(\text{conc}, (K[1], K[2], V_m[1], V_m[2])\bigr)$$

$$
= \begin{cases}
\dfrac{V_m[1]\text{conc}}{K[1]+\text{conc}} & \text{if} \quad \text{state} = \text{treated} \\[3mm]
\dfrac{V_m[2]\text{conc}}{K[2]+\text{conc}} & \text{if} \quad \text{state} = \text{untreated}
\end{cases}
\tag{8.1}
$$

In total, four parameters are used in the mean function because both K and V_m are assumed to vary from treatment to treatment. We can write the right-hand side more concisely as

$$\frac{V_m[\text{state}]\text{conc}}{K[\text{state}] + \text{conc}}$$

where we use the brackets (state) after parameters that vary as the grouping/treatment variable state changes. This is the most general model in the sense that the grouping is reflected in all parameters of the model. In Section 8.2, we will show how to simplify the model by collapsing parameters that do not differ between treatments.

8.1.1 Using nls()

The model given in Equation (8.1) is specified as follows using nls().

```
> Puromycin.m1 <- nls(rate ~ Vm[state] *
+     conc/(K[state] + conc), data = Puromycin,
+     start = list(K = c(0.1, 0.1),
+         Vm = c(200, 200)))
```

Using nls() is quite similar to our previous use of the function except for the use of the square brackets (with the grouping variable inside) to indicate the grouping: The construction Vm[state] means that the parameter V_m changes every time the level in the factor state changes, so we get two V_m parameters. Similarly, there are two K parameters (K[state]). The grouping variable between the square brackets can either be a factor (as in the example above) or a numeric vector (different numbers denote different groups). The use of square brackets does not work with self-starter functions.

The summary output is shown below.

```
> summary(Puromycin.m1)

Formula: rate ~ Vm[state] * conc/(K[state] + conc)

Parameters:
     Estimate Std. Error t value Pr(>|t|)
K1  6.412e-02  7.877e-03   8.141 1.29e-07 ***
K2  4.771e-02  8.281e-03   5.761 1.50e-05 ***
```

```
Vm1 2.127e+02  6.608e+00  32.185  < 2e-16 ***
Vm2 1.603e+02  6.896e+00  23.242 2.04e-15 ***
---
Signif. codes:  0 '***' 0.001 '**' 0.01 '*' 0.05 '.' 0.1 ' ' 1

Residual standard error: 10.4 on 19 degrees of freedom

Number of iterations to convergence: 7
Achieved convergence tolerance: 1.563e-06
```

This approach for fitting multiple curves is also described for another example in Venables and Ripley (2002a, Chapter 8), where a dataset with 21 curves is considered.

8.1.2 Using gnls()

The function gnls() (in the package nlme) provides a different interface for specifying grouping structures: The specification of the grouping is separated from the specification of the mean function. The additional argument params allows the user to specify parameter models for the parameters in the mean function. Otherwise the specification of gnls() is very similar to how it is done for nls().

```
> Puromycin.m2 <- gnls(rate ~ Vm *
+    conc/(K + conc), data = Puromycin,
+    start = list(Vm = c(200, 200),
+        K = c(0.1, 0.1)), params = list(Vm ~
+        state - 1, K ~ state -
+        1))
```

The list supplied to params contains a component related to each parameter. For the parameter V_m, the component is Vm~ state-1, which should be interpreted in much the same way as the following lm call, lm(a~state-1), fitting a one-way ANOVA structure in a parameterisation with no intercept term; that is, there will be a parameter for each group/treatment level (Dalgaard, 2002, Chapter 10). The same applies for the specification of the parameter model of K. The same starting values as used in the nls() call in Subsection 8.1.1 above are supplied.

The summary output from the gnls() fit is also obtained using the summary method.

```
> summary(Puromycin.m2)

Generalized nonlinear least squares fit
  Model: rate ~ Vm * conc/(K + conc)
  Data: Puromycin
       AIC       BIC     logLik
```

```
178.6001 184.2776 -84.30006
```

```
Coefficients:
                    Value Std.Error  t-value
Vm.statetreated   212.68374  6.608094 32.18534
Vm.stateuntreated 160.28005  6.896014 23.24242
K.statetreated      0.06412  0.007877  8.14053
K.stateuntreated    0.04771  0.008281  5.76105
                  p-value
Vm.statetreated         0
Vm.stateuntreated       0
K.statetreated          0
K.stateuntreated        0
```

```
 Correlation:
                  Vm.sttt Vm.sttn K.sttt
Vm.stateuntreated 0.000
K.statetreated    0.765   0.000
K.stateuntreated  0.000   0.777   0.000
```

```
Standardized residuals:
       Min          Q1         Med          Q3
-1.32632750 -0.52742160 -0.06890301  0.51295803
       Max
 2.44557124
```

```
Residual standard error: 10.40003
Degrees of freedom: 23 total; 19 residual
```

The results are very similar to the results based on Puromycin.m1, and the explanation given in Subsection 6.1.1 also applies here. The fitting function gnls() provides greater flexibility than nls() for analysis of grouped data, and it is also possible to use self-starter functions.

8.1.3 Using nlsList()

The function nlsList() (in the package nlme) partitions the data according to a grouping variable, and therefore it can also be used for fitting grouped data.

We use the self-starter function SSmicmen() followed by "|" and then the grouping factor.

```
> Puromycin.m3 <- nlsList(rate ~
+     SSmicmen(conc, Vm, K) | state,
+     data = Puromycin)
```

The argument `pool`, which we did not specify for `Puromycin.m3`, can be added to control whether or not the pooled standard error across groups should be used to calculate estimated standard errors. The default setting is `TRUE`, which results in a model fit identical to the fits in the previous two subsections. If the mean function is specified explicitly (without using a self-starter function), starting values for only one group have to be supplied, as they will be used as starting values for all groups.

Alternatively, the grouping structure can be specified explicitly first using the function `groupedData()` (Pinheiro and Bates, 2000, Section 3.2). Below we denote the grouped data object resulting from using `groupedData()` by `Puromycin2`.

```
> Puromycin2 <- groupedData(rate ~
+     conc | state, data = Puromycin)
```

The two arguments are a formula enhanced with "|" to indicate the grouping variable and the name of the dataset that contains the variables. The next step is to fit the model, supplying the generated grouped data object in the `data` argument in `nlsList()`.

```
> Puromycin.m4 <- nlsList(rate ~
+     SSmicmen(conc, a, b), data = Puromycin2)
```

The following methods can be applied to an `nlsList()` fit: `coef`, `fitted`, `plot` (residual plot), `predict` (predicted values), and `summary`.

8.2 Model reduction and parameter models

For grouped data, we distinguish between two situations. Interest lies in:

- comparing entire groups (e.g., is there any difference between two treatments in the `Puromycin` dataset?)
- comparing specific features/parameters between the groups

Subsection 8.2.1 shows how to compare groups, and Subsection 8.2.2 shows a series of more specific comparisons.

8.2.1 Comparison of entire groups

Let us consider the dataset `Puromycin` again. Looking at the plot in Fig. 8.1, there appears to be a difference between the treated and untreated groups: Treatment with the antibiotic puromycin results in a higher upper limit for the enzymatic reaction rate, so there seems to be a difference between the two treatments. Therefore we proceed to test the null hypothesis that the two parameters K and V_m do not differ between the two groups. The hypothesis can be formulated in terms of the parameters as follows.

$$K(\text{treated}) = K(\text{untreated}) \quad \text{and} \quad V_m(\text{treated}) = V_m(\text{untreated})$$

In order to do so, we need two model fits: one fit where both parameters in the Michaelis-Menten model vary from group to group and another fit where both parameters are assumed to be identical for the two groups. The model with varying parameters was already fitted in Subsections 8.1.1, 8.1.2, and 8.1.3, so we only need to fit the model assuming common parameters for both groups. This model is easily fitted, as we just leave out the grouped variable from the right-hand side of the model formula and modify the list of starting values accordingly.

```
> Puromycin.m5 <- nls(rate ~ Vm *
+     conc/(K + conc), data = Puromycin,
+     start = list(K = 0.1, Vm = 200))
```

In order to compare the two models, we use the F-test as it was defined in Subsection 7.5.2. The **anova** method provides a convenient way of obtaining the F-test of the null hypothesis.

```
> anova(Puromycin.m5, Puromycin.m1)

Analysis of Variance Table

Model 1: rate ~ Vm * conc/(K + conc)
Model 2: rate ~ Vm[state] * conc/(K[state] + conc)
  Res.Df Res.Sum Sq Df Sum Sq F value
1     21     7276.5
2     19     2055.1  2 5221.5  24.138
      Pr(>F)
1
2 6.075e-06 ***
---
Signif. codes:  0 '***' 0.001 '**' 0.01 '*' 0.05 '.' 0.1 ' ' 1
```

The null hypothesis is rejected with a p-value of 6.07e-06, indicating that the two groups are indeed very different.

8.2.2 Comparison of specific parameters

In this subsection, we consider a more elaborate approach where we only compare one parameter across groups at a time. Let us continue using the dataset Puromycin. In the previous subsection, we established that there is a difference between the treatments, but is it a difference in the parameter K or in the parameter V_m, or in both parameters? To be able to examine these questions, we need to use parameter models. Nonlinear regression models for grouped data give rise to model formulations for each parameter in the mean function. Take as an example the model fit Puromycin.m1 from Subsection 8.1.1. The two parameters K and V_m differ between groups, and therefore we can write the corresponding parameter models as follows:

$K \sim$ state
$V_m \sim$ state

Similarly, the model fit Puromycin.m5 corresponds to the following parameter models:

$K \sim 1$
$V_m \sim 1$

The parameter models above imply that there are common K and V_m parameters for both treatment groups. The two sets of parameter models listed above are the extremes where either all or none of the parameters in the mean function are shared across groups. Two other sets of parameter models can be envisaged for the Michaelis-Menten model fitted to the Puromycin dataset. The following parameter models assume different K and common V_m:

$K \sim$ state
$V_m \sim 1$

Finally, the parameter models below correspond to common K and different V_m:

$K \sim 1$
$V_m \sim$ state

These models are useful if we only want to compare one parameter across groups at a time. As already mentioned, Fig. 8.1 indicates that the upper limits (that is, the parameter V_m) differ between the treated and untreated groups. To examine whether or not a statistical test can confirm this impression, we fit the model corresponding to the null hypothesis $V_m(\text{treated}) = V_m(\text{untreated})$ with the aim of comparing it to the model fit Puromycin.m1. The model fit is obtained using nls() with the square brackets formulation introduced in Subsection 8.1.1.

```
> Puromycin.m6 <- nls(rate ~ Vm *
+     conc/(K[state] + conc), data = Puromycin,
+     start = list(K = c(0.1, 0.1),
+         Vm = 200))
```

The F-test is once more obtained using the anova method.

```
> anova(Puromycin.m6, Puromycin.m1)
```

```
Analysis of Variance Table


Model 1: rate ~ Vm * conc/(K[state] + conc)
Model 2: rate ~ Vm[state] * conc/(K[state] + conc)
  Res.Df Res.Sum Sq Df Sum Sq F value
1     20     4815.4
2     19     2055.1  1 2760.4  25.521
      Pr(>F)
1
2 7.082e-05 ***
---
Signif. codes:  0 '***' 0.001 '**' 0.01 '*' 0.05 '.' 0.1 ' ' 1
```

Thus we can safely conclude that the upper limits are different for the two treatments. Similarly, we can test the null hypothesis $H_0 : K(\text{treated}) = K(\text{untreated})$ by means of an F-test once we have fitted the corresponding model.

```
> Puromycin.m7 <- nls(rate ~ Vm[state] *
+     conc/(K + conc), data = Puromycin,
+     start = list(K = 0.1, Vm = c(200,
+         200))))
```

Again the anova method produces the results of the F-test.

```
> anova(Puromycin.m7, Puromycin.m1)

Analysis of Variance Table

Model 1: rate ~ Vm[state] * conc/(K + conc)
Model 2: rate ~ Vm[state] * conc/(K[state] + conc)
  Res.Df Res.Sum Sq Df  Sum Sq F value
1     20    2240.89
2     19    2055.05  1  185.84  1.7182
   Pr(>F)
1
2 0.2056
```

The p-value is 0.206, and we cannot reject the null hypothesis. This implies that the substrate concentration needed for the enzyme reaction rate to reach the level halfway between 0 and the upper limit is independent of the treatment, so the model fit Puromycin.m1 can be simplified to Puromycin.m7. The summary output for the final model fit Puromycin.m7 is shown below.

```
> summary(Puromycin.m7)

Formula: rate ~ Vm[state] * conc/(K + conc)
```

```
Parameters:
     Estimate Std. Error t value Pr(>|t|)
K      0.05797    0.00591   9.809 4.37e-09 ***
Vm1 208.63004    5.80399  35.946  < 2e-16 ***
Vm2 166.60408    5.80743  28.688  < 2e-16 ***
---
Signif. codes:  0 '***' 0.001 '**' 0.01 '*' 0.05 '.' 0.1 ' ' 1

Residual standard error: 10.59 on 20 degrees of freedom

Number of iterations to convergence: 7
Achieved convergence tolerance: 1.373e-06
```

The size of the difference between the upper limits, which we know is significantly different from 0, is roughly 42 counts/min/min. The common estimate of K is 0.058.

8.3 Common control

It may happen that a special type of grouped data occurs where the response values for a particular predictor value (typically 0) are not measured for each group but instead are measured separately and intended to serve as a common control for all other groups. We illustrate this situation through an example.

The dataset G.aparine originates from Cabanne et al. (1999). The experiment was designed to measure the effect of two formulations of the herbicide phenmedipham, which is a herbicide that does not move around in the plant, only exerting its effect where it hits the plants. Herbicide formulation 1 is the herbicide phenmedipham sprayed alone and herbicide formulation 2 is phenmedipham sprayed with an adjuvant that should enhance the effect. The test plant used was cleavers (*Galium aparine*). The same ten nonzero doses were used for both formulations, with ten replicates per dose. In addition, there were taken 20 replicates of the untreated control (dose equal to 0). The data are shown in Fig. 8.2 using xyplot().

```
> xyplot(drymatter ~ dose | as.factor(treatment),
+     data = G.aparine, xlab = "Dose (g/ha)",
+     ylab = "Dry matter (mg/pot)")
```

Cabanne et al. (1999) use the four-parameter log-logistic model introduced in Equation (1.6) in Section 1.3 to describe how drymatter changes with dose:

$$f\big(\text{dose}, (b, c, d, e)\big) = c + \frac{d - c}{1 + \exp(b(\log(\text{dose}) - \log(e)))} \tag{8.2}$$

Due to the common control measurements, there need to be some restrictions on the parameters. The upper limit is mainly determined by the common

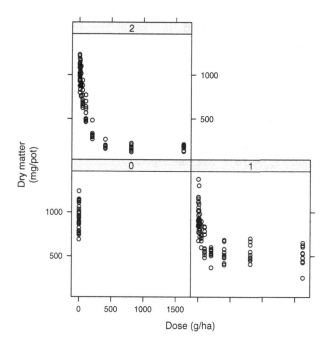

Fig. 8.2. Conditional scatter plot of the dose-response curves in the dataset G.aparine.

control measurements (shown in the bottom left window in Fig. 8.2), and therefore there is no point in assuming varying upper limits (the parameter d) across the two herbicide formulations. The remaining parameters b, c, and e can easily vary from formulation to formulation.

Before proceeding to fit the model, we need to do a little manipulation because the control measurements are grouped separately. They have their own values of the variable treatment equal to 0 (which was utilised in creating the plot in Fig. 8.2). This is useful for indicating that the control measurements form a separate group, which should not be used repeatedly as control measurements for each of the remaining groups, as that approach would illegally augment the dataset. However, it is not useful for a model fitting. For this purpose, it is convenient to assign the control measurements to one of the remaining groups. This is done in the following two R lines, where we define a new factor treatment2 inside the data frame G.aparine.

```
> G.aparine$treatment2 <- factor(G.aparine$treatment)
> levels(G.aparine$treatment2) <- c("1",
+      "1", "2")
```

The new factor `treatment2` is based on the grouping variable `treatment`. This means that after executing the first line the factor `treatment2` will have the levels 0, 1, and 2. In the second line, we change that: The `levels<-` replacement method is applied to change the levels into 1, 1, and 2, in effect collapsing the groups 0 and 1 into a single group. The choice of collapsing groups 0 and 1 rather than 0 and 2 is arbitrary, but the resulting model fit will be the same for both choices.

Now, we are ready to fit the model using `nls()` with the grouped-data specification outlined in Subsection 8.1.1.

```
> G.aparine.m1 <- nls(drymatter ~
+    c[treatment2] + (d - c[treatment2])/(1 +
+        exp(b[treatment2] * (log(dose) -
+            log(e[treatment2])))),
+    data = G.aparine, start = list(b = c(2,
+        2), c = c(500, 100), d = 1000,
+        e = c(50, 100)))
```

The parameters b, c, and e vary from one herbicide formulation to the other (indicated by the square brackets `[treatment2]`), whereas the parameter d is constant. The summary of the resulting model fit is shown below.

```
> summary(G.aparine.m1)
```

```
Formula: drymatter ~ c[treatment2] +
    (d - c[treatment2])/(1 + exp(b[treatment2] *
    (log(dose) - log(e[treatment2]))))
```

```
Parameters:
   Estimate Std. Error t value Pr(>|t|)
b1   1.6129     0.3462   4.659 5.33e-06 ***
b2   1.7510     0.2303   7.603 7.07e-13 ***
c1 509.5035    23.4379  21.738  < 2e-16 ***
c2 151.9164    27.2114   5.583 6.56e-08 ***
d  984.8883    12.7957  76.970  < 2e-16 ***
e1  50.8000     7.8465   6.474 5.58e-10 ***
e2  93.4466     8.1626  11.448  < 2e-16 ***
---
Signif. codes:  0 '***' 0.001 '**' 0.01 '*' 0.05 '.' 0.1 ' ' 1
```

```
Residual standard error: 111.4 on 233 degrees of freedom
```

```
Number of iterations to convergence: 7
Achieved convergence tolerance: 9.927e-06
```

The output shows that as expected only one upper limit (the parameter d) is estimated, whereas the remaining three parameters are estimated for each of the two formulations.

So it is possible to handle common control measurements by specifying the right model, using a common parameter across the grouping for the aspect of the model determined by the control measurement.

8.4 Prediction

Prediction for the grouped data situation proceeds in much the same way as outlined for a single curve in Subsection 2.2.3. We return to the dataset Puromycin to illustrate the concepts. We begin by defining the vector of predictor values; that is, concentrations.

```
> concValues <- with(Puromycin, seq(min(conc),
+     max(conc), length.out = 10))
> concValues

 [1] 0.02 0.14 0.26 0.38 0.50 0.62 0.74
 [8] 0.86 0.98 1.10
```

Similarly, we construct the grouping vector by extracting the group levels from the factor variable state.

```
> stateVal1 <- levels(Puromycin$state)
> stateVal1

[1] "treated"    "untreated"
```

Then we use the function expand.grid() to create the appropriate data frame containing both concentrations and grouping information.

```
> csValues1 <- expand.grid(conc = concValues,
+     state = stateVal1)
> csValues1

   conc      state
1  0.02    treated
2  0.14    treated
3  0.26    treated
4  0.38    treated
5  0.50    treated
6  0.62    treated
7  0.74    treated
8  0.86    treated
9  0.98    treated
10 1.10    treated
11 0.02  untreated
12 0.14  untreated
13 0.26  untreated
```

```
14 0.38 untreated
15 0.50 untreated
16 0.62 untreated
17 0.74 untreated
18 0.86 untreated
19 0.98 untreated
20 1.10 untreated
```

Finally, the `predict` method produces the requested predictions based on the final model fit obtained in Subsection 8.2.2.

```
> predict(Puromycin.m7, csValues1)

 [1]   53.51423 147.53721 170.59315
 [4]  181.01489 186.95393 190.79057
 [7]  193.47329 195.45463 196.97784
[10]  198.18535  42.73445 117.81765
[13]  136.22925 144.55166 149.29435
[16]  152.35815 154.50047 156.08269
[19]  157.29907 158.26334
```

The result is a vector of length $2 \cdot 10 = 20$; that is, ten predicted values for each group. If we only want predicted values for one particular group, then we still need to define the grouping vector as a factor. For instance, if we only want predicted values for the group "untreated", then the grouping vector has to be defined as follows:

```
> stateVal2 <- factor("untreated",
+     levels = c("treated", "untreated"))
> stateVal2

[1] untreated
Levels: treated untreated
```

The vector `stateVal2` has length 1, only containing the character string "untreated", but through the argument `levels` it is ensured that it is defined as a factor with two levels: "treated" and "untreated". In the following construction of the data frame, it will be replicated appropriately; that is, repeated for each element in the vector `concValues`.

```
> csValues2 <- data.frame(conc = concValues,
+     state = stateVal2)
> csValues2

  conc     state
1 0.02 untreated
2 0.14 untreated
3 0.26 untreated
```

```
4   0.38 untreated
5   0.50 untreated
6   0.62 untreated
7   0.74 untreated
8   0.86 untreated
9   0.98 untreated
10  1.10 untreated
```

The predict method can be applied in the same way as before.

```
> predict(Puromycin.m1, csValues2)
[1]   47.3444 119.5430 135.4296 142.4018
[5] 146.3188 148.8279 150.5725 151.8559
[9] 152.8395 153.6175
```

The result is a vector of length 10 that is identical to the last ten predicted values obtained above using csValues1.

8.5 Nonlinear mixed models

In this section, we introduce nonlinear mixed models by means of an example. It is intended to be an appetizer only. Pinheiro and Bates (2000) provides a comprehensive introduction to all the facets of nonlinear mixed model analysis in **R**.

Nellemann et al. (2003) carried out experiments to assess the in vitro and in vivo effects of the fungicides procymidone and vinclozolin. We will only consider the data obtained from the in vitro assessment of vinclozolin. The data were obtained using an androgen receptor reporter gene assay, which was repeated six times (on different days). Each assay resulted in concentration-response data with nine concentrations (in μM) of the fungicide, and the response measured was chemiluminescence (in luminescence units), so the same nine concentrations were used in all six assays. However, in one assay, only eight concentrations were used. It is expected that there will be some variation between the experiments (interassay variation), which may partly be due to varying efficiency from assay to assay, but it may also be due to other conditions that vary from day to day. Thus we expect that there are two sources of variation in the data: variation between the measurements within each assay (this is the measurement error) and variation between assays.

The data are available in **R** in the package drc as the data frame vinclozolin, and they are shown in Fig. 8.3. The variables in the data frame are the predictor variable conc, the response variable effect, and the grouping variable exper. The concentration-response pattern in the data is apparent from Fig. 8.3.

```
> xyplot(effect ~ conc | exper, data = vinclozolin,
+     xlab = expression(paste("Concentration (",
+         mu, "M)")), ylab = "Luminescence (LU)")
```

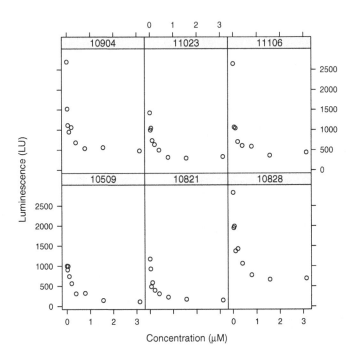

Fig. 8.3. Conditional scatter plot of the dose-response curves in the dataset vin-clozolin.

Following Nellemann et al. (2003), we will use the three-parameter log-logistic model given by the mean function:

$$f\big(\text{conc}, (b, d, e)\big) = \frac{d}{1 + \left(\frac{\text{conc}}{e}\right)^{b}} \tag{8.3}$$

We start out by fitting such a model to the data from each assay separately using nls(). There are several reasons for taking this route. One reason is that in many cases it is easier to fit the model to the individual curves than to the collection of curves, and this approach also provides good starting values for the model involving all curves. In general, it may be a good idea to build a model for grouped data on the basis of models for the individual groups.

We anticipate interassay variation, but the question is in which parameters this variation manifests itself. It can happen that there is a lot of variation across assays for all parameters in the model function, but more often it only shows up in a few or even a single parameter.

The individual assay data are fitted below using `nls()`, supplying sensible starting values.

```
> LL3.formula <- effect ~ d/(1 +
+     exp(b * (log(conc) - log(e))))
> vinclozolin.e1.m <- nls(LL3.formula,
+     data = vinclozolin, subset = exper ==
+         10509, start = list(b = 1,
+         d = 1000, e = 0.26))
> vinclozolin.e2.m <- nls(LL3.formula,
+     data = vinclozolin, subset = exper ==
+         10821, start = list(b = 1,
+         d = 1200, e = 0.074))
> vinclozolin.e3.m <- nls(LL3.formula,
+     data = vinclozolin, subset = exper ==
+         10828, start = list(b = 1,
+         d = 2800, e = 0.15))
> vinclozolin.e4.m <- nls(LL3.formula,
+     data = vinclozolin, subset = exper ==
+         10904, start = list(b = 1,
+         d = 2700, e = 0.03))
> vinclozolin.e5.m <- nls(LL3.formula,
+     data = vinclozolin, subset = exper ==
+         11023, start = list(b = 1,
+         d = 1400, e = 0.14))
> vinclozolin.e6.m <- nls(LL3.formula,
+     data = vinclozolin, subset = exper ==
+         11106, start = list(b = 0.5,
+         d = 2600, e = 0.02))
```

Note how we initially define a model formula (`LL3.formula`) and then use it repeatedly in the six model fits. The following **R** lines create a plot of the data and the fitted concentration-response curves.

```
> plot(effect ~ conc, data = vinclozolin,
+     pch = as.numeric(exper), log = "x",
+     xlim = c(1e-04, 10), xlab = expression(paste
+         ("Concentration(", mu, "M)")), ylab = "Luminescence(LU)")
> concVec <- exp(seq(log(1e-04),
+     log(10), length.out = 50))
> lines(concVec, predict(vinclozolin.e1.m,
+     data.frame(conc = concVec)),
+     lty = 2)
> lines(concVec, predict(vinclozolin.e2.m,
```

```
+      data.frame(conc = concVec)),
+      lty = 3)
> lines(concVec, predict(vinclozolin.e3.m,
+      data.frame(conc = concVec)),
+      lty = 4)
> lines(concVec, predict(vinclozolin.e4.m,
+      data.frame(conc = concVec)),
+      lty = 5)
> lines(concVec, predict(vinclozolin.e5.m,
+      data.frame(conc = concVec)),
+      lty = 6)
> lines(concVec, predict(vinclozolin.e6.m,
+      data.frame(conc = concVec)),
+      lty = "3313")
```

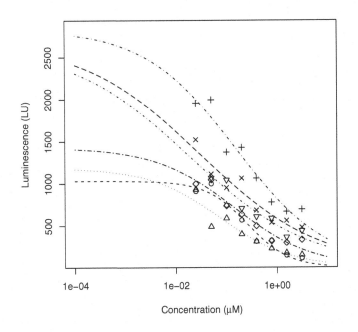

Fig. 8.4. Fitted dose-response curves based on individual fits of the three-parameter log-logistic model for each assay in the dataset `vinclozolin` (dashed lines). The unusual line type specification for the sixth assay is needed to avoid getting a solid line (read more on the help page of `par`).

The resulting plot is shown in Fig. 8.4, indicating that the interassay variation is by far most pronounced at concentration 0; that is, in the variation in the upper limit (the parameter d). Figure 8.4 shows that for each assay the three-parameter log-logistic model roughly speaking captures the assay-specific concentration-response trend. However, the real interest lies in the overall dose-response trend (sometimes called the population trend), which is the trend adjusted for assay-specific distortions or shifts.

The previous sections and chapters have considered nonlinear regression models assuming one single source of randomness: the error attached to each individual measurement. As we have seen in Fig. 8.4, for a group of assays, the variation between assays also needs to be considered. We can think of this variation as being derived by minute unobservable changes in the environment of the assay that occur at random. In a nonlinear mixed-model approach, this randomness is quantified in terms of random effects. In Equation (8.3), there are three parameters (b, d, and e), but for each individual assay, we only observe a concentration-response curve where each parameter is distorted by some positive or negative quantities: $b + \delta_1$, $d + \delta_2$, and $e + \delta_3$. The quantities δ_1, δ_2, and δ_3 are the random effects, which explain the part of the variation stemming from unobservable sources such as changes in environmental conditions. Consequently, there will be different random effects in play for different assays, but still it is usually assumed that random effects for the same parameter from different assays follow the same normal distribution with mean 0 and some unknown variance parameter, which is often called a variance component. This means that a nonlinear mixed model is a nonlinear regression model that has been extended by allowing some or all of the parameters to vary randomly across groups in order to account for the variation between groups. Another consequence of introducing random effects is that all measurements within a group are correlated, reflecting the fact that they all share the same experimental conditions.

In contrast, the parameters b, d, and e are called the fixed effects or fixed-effects parameters, as they remain constant across the groups. The fixed-effects parameters explain the part of the variation in the data that is largely determined by the recorded predictor variables. In the case of the dataset vinclozolin, the systematic concentration-response trend is governed largely by the fungicide concentration (the predictor variable). The fixed-effect parameters should be viewed as average or population parameter values.

As we are considering grouped data, it is natural to formulate parameter models similar to what was done in Section 8.2.2, but we will extend the specification by considering parameter models for both the fixed effects and the random effects.

The parameter models for the fixed effects are given below.

```
b ~ 1
d ~ 1
e ~ 1
```

There is only one b, one d, and one e, as the six assays are repeated without changing the experimental design. The parameter models for the random-effects part of the model are then specified having our initial individual analysis results in mind.

d ~ exper

This means that random effects are only assigned to the parameter d (the upper limit) but not to the parameters b and e.

The random effects are assumed to be normally distributed with mean 0 and an unknown variance σ^2_{exper}, so the introduction of random effects means that there are two layers of variation, both of which are described by means of normal distributions. Therefore such a model is often called a hierarchical model. Inclusion of random effects according to the parameter model above means that one additional parameter has to be estimated, namely the variance component σ^2_{exper}, reflecting the variation exhibited in the six random effects.

Another way to think about the model is to imagine that for each assay or group a random parameter determining the upper limit was sampled from a normal distribution with mean d and variance σ^2_{exper}. Thus, in a hypothetical situation with many assays available, the average upper limit across the assays would be close to d, and we would expect roughly 95% of the assays to have upper limits within a distance of $2\sigma_{exper}$ from d.

Nonlinear mixed models can be fitted in **R** using the fitting function nlme() in the package nlme (Pinheiro and Bates, 2000, Chapter 7). The parameter models above translate into the following specification of nlme():

```
> vinclozolin.m1 <- nlme(effect ~
+    d/(1 + exp(b * (log(conc) -
+       log(e)))), fixed = list(b ~
+    1, d ~ 1, e ~ 1), random = d ~
+    1 | exper, start = c(1, 1000,
+    0.1), data = vinclozolin)
```

We assess the model fit by adding the fitted concentration-response curve to the plot shown in Fig. 8.4.

```
> lines(concVec, predict(vinclozolin.m1,
+    data.frame(conc = concVec),
+    level = 0), lty = 1, lwd = 3)
```

The argument level determines which kinds of predictions should be returned. The level 0 corresponds to the average trend or population trend, which is what we are interested in here. Figure 8.5 shows that the population concentration-response trend based on the six assays lies somewhere in the middle between the six individual assay-specific concentration-response trends.

The summary of the model fit is as usual obtained using summary.

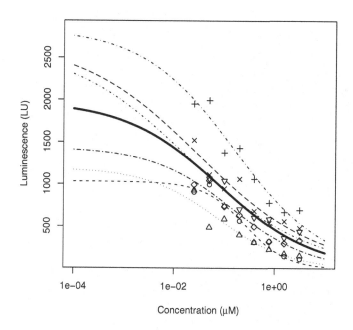

Fig. 8.5. Fitted dose-response curves based on individual fits of the three-parameter log-logistic model for each assay (the dashed lines) and the fitted dose-response curve based on a nonlinear mixed-model analysis of the dataset `vinclozolin` (solid).

```
> summary(vinclozolin.m1)

Nonlinear mixed-effects model fit by maximum likelihood
  Model: effect ~ d/(1 + exp(b * (log(conc) - log(e))))
  Data: vinclozolin
        AIC       BIC    logLik
   715.5204 725.3719 -352.7602

Random effects:
 Formula: d ~ 1 | exper
                d Residual
StdDev: 695.3775 150.9623

Fixed effects: list(b ~ 1, d ~ 1, e ~ 1)
       Value Std.Error DF   t-value p-value
b     0.4654   0.03896 45 11.945080       0
d 1976.4209 298.62209 45  6.618468       0
```

```
e    0.0793   0.01483 45  5.349841      0
Correlation:
  b      d
d -0.051
e  0.529 -0.145
```

```
Standardized Within-Group Residuals:
      Min           Q1           Med          Q3
-1.83842038  -0.58871949  -0.06161384   0.54652837
      Max
 2.07902662
```

```
Number of Observations: 53
Number of Groups: 6
```

The summary output contains:

- the model specification together with some measures for model selection
- the estimated variance components
- the estimated fixed-effects parameters (the three parameters in Equation (8.3))
- the five-number summary of the residuals
- the number of observations and the number of groups

The nonlinear mixed-model analysis has succinctly summarised the six assays, both yielding estimates for the parameters in the three-parameter log-logistic model that are of direct interest in this example (Nellemann et al., 2003) and giving an idea about the interassay variability in this kind of experiment, which is roughly 4–5 times as large as the within-assay variability.

To extract the estimated fixed-effects parameters and the estimated variance component and residual variance (and corresponding standard deviations), the functions fixef() and VarCorr(), respectively, can be used. The estimated fixed-effects parameters and standard deviations with the accompanying approximate confidence intervals can be obtained using intervals().

Apart from the predict and summary methods already used, there is a plot method for displaying the residual plot. The residuals can be extracted directly using the residuals method. We refer to Pinheiro and Bates (2000, Appendix B) for a complete overview of the available functions and methods.

In practice, there often occurs both a grouping variable, which we need to use to account for between-group variation, and a treatment variable (or even several such variables), which is of primary interest. This means that the parameter models will have to reflect the grouping structure both in the fixed effects and the random effects (see Exercise 8.5 for an example).

Exercises

8.1. Fit an appropriate grouped data model to the dataset S.alba introduced in Section 1.3.

8.2. The asymptotic regression model can be used to describe growth. The corresponding mean function is defined as follows:

$$f\big(x, (a, b, c)\big) = a + (b - a)(1 - \exp(-cx))$$

Fit the model to the dataset methionine.

8.3. Obtain the predicted value for a dose value of 500 based on the model fit G.aparine.m1.

8.4. Fit the three-parameter log-logistic model to the dataset vinclozolin, but this time using a model where random effects are assigned to all three parameters. Use the summary output for the resulting model fit to decide the parameter for which to omit the corresponding random effects. Fit the simplified model. Use the anova method to confirm that there is no evidence in the data against the simplified model.

8.5. Nielsen et al. (2004) consider a nonlinear mixed-model analysis of the dataset provided in the data frame spinach. Consider the following parameter models based on a four-parameter log-logistic model for the fixed and random effects:

Fixed effects
    b ~ HERBICIDE
    c ~ HERBICIDE
    d ~ HERBICIDE
    e ~ HERBICIDE

Random effects
    c ~ CURVE
    d ~ CURVE

Fit the corresponding nonlinear mixed model using nlme().

Appendix A: Datasets and Models

Table A.1. Models considered in this book.

Model	Page
Antoine	56
Beverton-Holt	2, 106
Biexponential	87
Brain-Cousens	58, 71, 108
Clapeyron	56
Demodulator	48
Deriso	106
Exponential decay	24, 31
Hockey stick	41
Hyperbolic	4, 35
Logistic	70, 101
Log-logistic (4 parameters)	5, 60, 118
Log-logistic (3 parameters)	58
Michaelis-Menten	9, 30
Monoexponential	108
Ricker	78, 106
Shepherd	106
Verhulst	70

Table **A.2.** Datasets used in this book.

Discipline Name	Page	Package
Biology		
exp1	87	nlrwr
exp2	87	nlrwr
L.minor	9	nlrwr
Leaves	35	NRAIA
methionine	131	drc
RGRcurve	33	nlrwr
RScompetition	4, 45	drc
ScotsPine	108	nlrwr
Chemistry		
btb	35	nlrwr
Isom	53	NRAIA
sts	35	nlrwr
vapCO	56	nlrwr
Fisheries		
M.merluccius	2, 105	nlrwr
O.mykiss	91	drc, nlrwr
sockeye	78	nlrwr
Engineering		
Chwirut2	23	NISTnls
IQsig	48	nlrwr
Medicine		
heartrate	71	drc
Puromycin	109	datasets
wtloss	20	MASS
Toxicology		
G.aparine	118	drc
lettuce	57	drc
ryegrass	60	drc
S.alba	4	drc
secalonic	101	drc
spinach	131	drc
vinclozolin	123	drc
Other		
Indometh (pharmacokinetics)	71	datasets
segreg (energy consumption)	44	alr3
US.pop (population growth)	71	car

Appendix B: Self-starter Functions

Table B.1. Available self-starter functions for `nls()`.

Model	No. param.	Self-starter function *Mean function*
Biexponential	4	`SSbiexp(x, A1, lrc1, A2, lrc2)` $A1 \cdot \exp(-\exp(lrc1) \cdot x) + A2 \cdot \exp(-\exp(lrc2) \cdot x)$
Asymptotic regression	3	`SSasymp(x, Asym, R0, lrc)` $Asym + (R0 - Asym) \cdot \exp(-\exp(lrc)x)$
Asymptotic regression with offset	3	`SSasympOff(x, Asym, lrc, c0)` $Asym \cdot (1 - \exp(-\exp(lrc)(x - c0)))$
Asymptotic regression $(c0 = 0)$	2	`SSasympOrig(x, Asym, lrc)` $Asym \cdot (1 - \exp(-\exp(lrc)x))$
First-order compartment	3	`SSfol(x1, x2, lKe, lKa, lCl)` $x1 \cdot \exp(lKe + lKa - lCl)/(\exp(lKa) - \exp(lKe))$ $\cdot(\exp(-\exp(lKe)x2) - \exp(-\exp(lKa)x2))$
Gompertz	3	`SSgompertz(x, Asym, b2, b3)` $Asym \cdot \exp(-b2 \cdot b3^x)$
Logistic	4	`SSfpl(x, A, B, xmid, scal)` $A + (B - A)/(1 + \exp((xmid - x)/scal))$
Logistic $(A = 0)$	3	`SSlogis(x, Asym, xmid, scal)` $Asym/(1 + \exp((xmid - x)/scal))$
Michaelis-Menten	2	`SSmicmen(x, Vm, K)` $Vm \cdot x/(K + x)$
Weibull	4	`SSweibull(x, Asym, Drop, lrc, pwr)` $Asym - Drop \cdot \exp(-\exp(lrc) \cdot x^p wr)$

Appendix C: Packages and Functions

All the packages listed below will be available in the R session after installation of nlrwr from CRAN (http://cran.r-project.org) and subsequent loading (using library(nlrwr)).

Table C.1. Packages used in this book.

Package	Description
alr3	Methods and data to accompany Weisberg (2005)
car	Companion to Applied Regression
datasets	The R Datasets Package (in the R standard installation)
drc	Analysis of dose-response curve
HydroMe	Estimation of Soil Hydraulic Parameters from Experimental Data
lattice	Lattice Graphics
lmtest	Testing Linear Regression Models
MASS	Support software for Venables and Ripley (2002)
NISTnls	Nonlinear least-squares examples from NIST
nlme	Linear and Nonlinear Mixed Effects Models
nlrwr	Support package for this book
nls2	Nonlinear regression with brute force
nlstools	Tools for nonlinear regression diagnostics
NRAIA	Datasets from Bates and Watts (1988)
sandwich	Robust Covariance Matrix Estimators
stats	The R Stats Package (in the R standard installation)

Table **C.2.** Main functions used in this book.

Function	Package	Page
AIC()	stats	107
bartlett.test()	stats	65
bcSummary()	nlrwr	82
boxcox.nls()	nlrwr	82
coeftest()	lmtest	85
confint2()	nlrwr	99
delta.method()	alr3	100
deriv()	stats	40
getInitial()	stats	34
glm()	stats	19
gnls()	nlme	112
levene.test()	car	65
nlme()	nlme	128
nls()	stats	*All over the book!*
nls.control()	stats	52
nls2()	nls2	28
nlsBoot()	nlstools	97
nlsContourRSS()	nlstools	16
nlsList()	nlme	113
plotfit()	NRAIA (also in nlstools)	20
sandwich()	sandwich	84
selfStart()	stats	33
shapiro.test()	stats	69
xyplot()	lattice	6, 118, 123

References

Bailer, A. J. and Piegorsch, W. W. (2000). From quantal counts to mechanisms and systems: The past, present and future of biometrics in environmental toxicology. *Biometrics* **56**, 327–336.

Bates, D. M. and Chambers, J. M. (1992). *Statistical Models in S*, chapter 10 (Nonlinear Models). Chapman and Hall, Boca Raton, Fl.

Bates, D. M. and Watts, D. G. (1988). *Nonlinear Regression Analysis and Its Applications*. John Wiley and Sons, New York.

Beckon, W. N., Parkins, C., Maximovich, A., and Beckon, A. V. (2008). A general approach to modeling biphasic relationships. *Environ. Sci. Technol.* **42**, 1308–1314.

Box, G. E. P. and Cox, D. R. (1964). An analysis of transformations. *J. R. Stat. Soc. B* **26**, 211–246.

Brain, P. and Cousens, R. (1989). An equation to describe dose responses where there is stimulation of growth at low dose. *Weed Res.* **29**, 93–96.

Brazzale, A. (2005). hoa: An R package bundle for higher order likelihood inference. *R News* **5**, 20–27.

Burnham, K. P. and Anderson, D. R. (2002). *Model Selection and Multimodel Inference: A Practical Information-Theoretic Approach*. Springer, New York, second edition.

Cabanne, F., Gaudry, J. C., and Streibig, J. C. (1999). Influence of alkyl oleates on efficacy of phenmedipham applied as an acetone:water solution on *Galium aparine*. *Weed Res.* **39**, 57–67.

Cadima, E. L. (2003). *Fish Stock Assessment Manual*. Technical report, FAO Fisheries Department. ftp://ftp.fao.org/docrep/fao/006/x8498e/x8498e00.pdf.

Carroll, R. J. and Ruppert, D. (1984). Power transformations when fitting theoretical models to data. *J. Am. Stat. Assoc.* **79**, 321–328.

Carroll, R. J. and Ruppert, D. (1988). *Transformation and Weighting in Regression*. Chapman and Hall, New York.

Cedergreen, N., Andersen, L., Olesen, C. F., Spliid, H. H., and Streibig, J. C. (2005). Does the effect of herbicide pulse exposure on aquatic plants depend on K_{ow} or mode of action? *Aquat. Toxicol.* **72**, 261–271.

Cedergreen, N. and Madsen, T. V. (2002). Nitrogen uptake by the floating macrophyte *Lemna minor*. *New Phytol.* **155**, 285–292.

Cedergreen, N., Ritz, C., and Streibig, J. C. (2005). Improved empirical models describing hormesis. *Environ. Toxicol. Chem.* **24**, 3166–3172.

Christensen, M. G., Teicher, H. B., and Streibig, J. C. (2003). Linking fluorescence induction curve and biomass in herbicide screening. *Pest Management Science* **59**, 1303–1310.

Dalgaard, P. (2002). *Introductory Statistics with R*. Springer-Verlag, New York.

Ducharme, G. R. and Fontez, B. (2004). A smooth test of goodness-of-fit for growh curves and monotonic nonlinear regression models. *Biometrics* **60**, 977–986.

Environment Canada (2005). *Guidance Document on Statistical Methods for Environmental Toxicity Tests*. Environment Canada, Ottawa.

Fox, J. (2002). Nonlinear regression and nonlinear least squares. Appendix to *An R and S-PLUS Companion to Applied Regression*, Sage Publications, Ca.

Gong, X., Zeng, R., Luo, S., Yong, C., and Zheng, Q. (2004). Two new secalonic acids from *Aspergillus japonicus* and their allelopathic effects on higher plants. In *Proceedings of International Symposium on Allelopathy Research and Application, 27–29 April, Shanshui, Guangdong, China*, pages 209–217. Zongkai University of Agriculture and Technology, Guangzhou.

Hamilton, D. C. and Knop, O. (1998). Combining non-linear regressions that have unequal error variances and some parameters in common. *Appl. Statist.* **47**, 173–185.

Huet, S., Bouvier, A., Poursat, M.-A., and Jolivet, E. (2004). *Statistical Tools for Nonlinear Regression: A Practical Guide with S-PLUS and R Examples*. Springer-Verlag, New York, second edition.

Inderjit, Streibig, J. C., and Olofsdotter, M. (2002). Joint action of phenolic acid mixtures and its significance in allelopathy research. *Physiologia Plantarum* **114**, 422–428.

Jensen, J. E. (1993). Fitness of herbicide-resistant weed biotypes described by competition models. In *Proceedings of the 8th EWRS Symposium, 14–16 June, Braunschweig, Germany*, volume 1, pages 25–32. European Weed Research Society.

Kafadar, K. (1994). An application of nonlinear regression in research and development: A case study from the electronics industry. *Technometrics* **36**, 237–248.

Laberge, G., Ambus, P., Hauggaard-Nielsen, H., and Jensen, E. S. (2006). Stabilization and plant uptake of N from ^{15}N-labelled pea residue 16.5 years after incorporation in soil. *Soil Biol. Biochem.* **38**, 1998–2000.

McCullagh, P. and Nelder, J. A. (1989). *Generalized Linear Models.* Chapman and Hall, Boca Raton, Fl, second edition.

Motulsky, H. J. and Christopoulos, A. (2004). *Fitting Models to Biological Data Using Linear and Nonlinear Regression: A Practical Guide to Curve Fitting.* Oxford University Press, Oxford.

Murrell, P. (2006). *R Graphics.* Chapman and Hall, Boca Raton, Fl.

Nelder, J. A. (1991). Generalized linear models for enzyme-kinetic data. *Biometrics* **47**, 1605–1615.

Nellemann, C., Dalgaard, M., Lam, H. R., and Vinggaard, A. M. (2003). The combined effects of vinclozolin and procymidone do not deviate from expected additivity *in vitro* and *in vivo. Toxicol. Sci.* **71**, 251–262.

Nielsen, O. K., Ritz, C., and Streibig, J. C. (2004). Nonlinear mixed-model regression to analyze herbicide dose-response relationships. *Weed Technol.* **18**, 30–37.

NIST (National Institute of Standards and Technology) (1979). *Ultrasonic Reference Study Block (D. Chwirut).* Technical report. http://www.itl.nist.gov/div898/strd/nls/data/chwirut2.shtml.

OECD (Organisation for Economic Cooperation and Development) (2006b). *Current Approaches in the Statistical Analysis of Ecotoxicity Data: A Guidance to Application.* OECD Environment Health and Safety Publications, Series on Testing and Assessment, No. 54, Organisation for Economic Cooperation and Development, Paris.

OECD (Organisation for Economic Cooperation and Development) (2006a). *Current Approaches in the Statistical Analysis of Ecotoxicity Data: A Guidance to Application – Annexes.* OECD Environment Health and Safety Publications, Series on Testing and Assessment, No. 54, Organisation for Economic Cooperation and Development, Paris.

Pedersen, B. P., Neve, P., Andreasen, C., and Powles, S. (2007). Ecological fitness of a glyphosate-resistant *Lolium rigidum* population: Growth and seed production along a competition gradient. *Basic Appl. Ecol.* **8**, 258–268.

Pinheiro, J. C. and Bates, D. M. (2000). *Mixed-Effects Models in S and S-PLUS.* Springer-Verlag, New York.

Seber, G. A. F. and Wild, C. J. (1989). *Nonlinear Regression.* John Wiley and Sons, New York.

Streibig, J. C., Rudemo, M., and Jensen, J. E. (1993). Dose-response curves and statistical models. In Streibig, J. C. and Kudsk, P., editors, *Herbicide Bioassays*, pages 29–55, CRC Press, Boca Raton, Fl.

van der Vaart, A. W. (1998). *Asymptotic Statistics.* Cambridge University Press, Cambridge.

van Ewijk, P. H. and Hoekstra, J. A. (1993). Calculation of the EC50 and its confidence interval when subtoxic stimulus is present. *Ecotoxicology and Environmental Safety* **25**, 25–32.

Van Ness, H. C. and Abbott, M. (1997). *Perry's Chemical Engineers' Handbook*, chapter 4 (Thermodynamics). McGraw-Hill, seventh edition.

Venables, W. N. and Ripley, B. D. (2002a). *Modern Applied Statistics with S*. Springer, New York, fourth edition. ISBN 0-387-95457-0.

Venables, W. N. and Ripley, B. D. (2002b). Statistics Complements to Modern Applied Statistics with S (fourth edition).

Watkins, P. and Venables, W. N. (2006). Non-linear regression for optimising the separation of carboxylic acids. *R News* **6**, 2–7.

Weisberg, S. (2005). *Applied Linear Regression*. John Wiley and Sons, New York, third edition.

White, H. (1981). Consequences and detection of misspecifed nonlinear regression models. *J. Am. Stat. Assoc.* **76**, 419–433.

White, H. (1996). *Estimation, Inference and Specification Analysis*. Cambridge University Press, Cambridge.

Zeileis, A. (2006). Object-oriented computation of sandwich estimators. *J. Statist. Software* **16**, 1–16.

Zeileis, A. and Hothorn, T. (2002). Diagnostic checking in regression relationships. *R News* **2**, 7–10.

Index

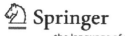

springer.com

A Modern Approach to Regression with R

Simon J. Sheather

This book focuses on tools and techniques for building regression models using real-world data and assessing their validity. The book contains a number of new real data sets from applications ranging from rating restaurants, rating wines, predicting newspaper circulation and magazine revenue, comparing the performance of NFL kickers, and comparing finalists in the Miss America pageant across states. One of the aspects of the book that sets it apart from many other regression books is that complete details are provided for each example. The book is aimed at first year graduate students in statistics and could also be used for a senior undergraduate class.

2009. Approx. 495 pp. (Springer Texts in Statistics) Hardcover
ISBN 978-0-387-09607-0

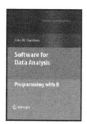

Software for Data Analysis
Programming with R

John M. Chambers

This book guides the reader through programming with R, beginning with simple interactive use and progressing by gradual stages, starting with simple functions. More advanced programming techniques can be added as needed, allowing users to grow into software contributors, benefiting their careers and the community. R packages provide a powerful mechanism for contributions to be organized and communicated.

2008. Approx. 510 pp. (Statistics and Computing) Hardcover
ISBN 978-0-387-75935-7

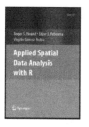

Applied Spatial Data Analysis with R

Roger S. Bivand, Edzer J. Pebesma, and Virgilio Gómez-Rubio

This book is divided into two basic parts, the first presenting R packages, functions, classes and methods for handling spatial data. The second part showcases more specialised kinds of spatial data analysis, including spatial point pattern analysis, interpolation and geostatistics, areal data analysis and disease mapping. The coverage of methods of spatial data analysis ranges from standard techniques to new developments, and the examples used are largely taken from the spatial statistics literature. All the examples can be run using R contributed packages available from the CRAN website, with code and additional data sets from the book's own website.

2008. Approx 400 pp. (Use R!) Softcover
ISBN 978-0-387-78170-9

Easy Ways to Order▶   Call: Toll-Free 1-800-SPRINGER • E-mail: orders-ny@springer.com • Write: Springer, Dept. S8113, PO Box 2485, Secaucus, NJ 07096-2485 • Visit: Your local scientific bookstore or urge your librarian to order.